AN INTRODUCTION TO THE WORK OF A MEDICAL EXAMINER

AN INTRODUCTION TO THE WORK OF A MEDICAL EXAMINER

From Death Scene to Autopsy Suite

JOHN J. MILETICH
AND
TIA LAURA LINDSTROM

Foreword by Cyril H. Wecht, M.D., J.D.

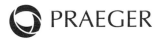 PRAEGER

AN IMPRINT OF ABC-CLIO, LLC
Santa Barbara, California • Denver, Colorado • Oxford, England

Library of Congress Cataloging-in-Publication Data

Miletich, John J.
　　An introduction to the work of a medical examiner : from death scene to autopsy suite / John J. Miletich and Tia Laura Lindstrom; foreword by Cyril H. Wecht.
　　　　p. cm.
　　Includes bibliographical references and index.
　　ISBN 978-0-275-99508-9 (hard copy : alk. paper) — ISBN 978-0-275-99509-6 (ebook)
　　1. Autopsy. 2. Forensic pathology. 3. Death—Causes. I. Lindstrom, Tia Laura. II. Title.
　　RA1063.4.M55 2010
　　614'.1—dc22　　　　2009048542

ISBN: 978-0-275-99508-9
EISBN: 978-0-275-99509-6

14　13　12　11　10　　　1　2　3　4　5

This book is also available on the World Wide Web as an eBook.
Visit www.abc-clio.com for details.

Praeger
An Imprint of ABC-CLIO, LLC

ABC-CLIO, LLC
130 Cremona Drive, P.O. Box 1911
Santa Barbara, California 93116-1911

This book is printed on acid-free paper ∞

Manufactured in the United States of America

To my sister, Margaret —JJM
For my husband, Kevin —TLL

CONTENTS

FOREWORD

———•◦•———

THE RAPID CREATION and expansion of forensic science programs in universities and colleges over the past two decades are unparalleled in the history of U.S. academia in modern times. There are now approximately 350 such curricula with varying areas of primary emphasis. Many high schools have also initiated forensic science courses, in a few instances spanning both semesters of a school year.

Contrary to popular opinion, this field of medical-legal specialization did not spring anew from television programs like *Quincy* and *CSI*. In fact, references to the application and utilization of scientific knowledge in the investigation of violent and suspicious deaths can be found in the chronicles of ancient civilizations thousands of years ago. Antistius, the great Roman physician, examined the body of Julius Caesar and determined that only one of the 23 knife wounds he sustained would have been fatal.

Loyal knights appointed by English Kings gave birth to the Coroner System in the twelfth century, and the Chinese put together an extensive set of guidelines ("The Washing of Wrongs") for such observations and procedures to be followed when dealing with puzzling deaths in the fourteenth century.

In the sixteenth century, Zacchia, physician to the Pope, authored a magnificent volume, *Questiones de Medicina Legalis*, in which he posed hundreds of specific contentious scenarios that he then analyzed and answered.

Following the Dark Ages, with the creation of institutions of higher learning throughout various parts of Europe, legal medicine and forensic science came to be an integral part of many medical school curricula. Numerous textbooks dealing with these subjects written in the nineteenth century continued to be revised and used by physicians and other scientists well into the twentieth century.

In more recent decades, beginning with the assassination of President John F. Kennedy and continuing until the present time with other famous and controversial cases—Robert F. Kennedy, Mary Jo Kopechne, Elvis Presley, Jean Harris, Sunny Von Bulow, Vincent Foster, the Waco Branch Davidian fire-shootout, O.J. Simpson, JonBenet Ramsey, Laci Peterson, Phil Spector, Anna Nicole and Daniel Smith, Michael Jackson, and many others—the American public has come to learn about the complex and extremely relevant roles played by a variety of forensic scientists in attempting to determine the cause and manner of death, the time and place of the fatal event, and occasionally, the analysis of bodily and environmental materials that can lead to the actual identification of the assailant.

Of course, all the *CSI* and other television series with a similar theme have fueled the general public's interest and whetted the intellectual appetite of millions of people regarding forensic science. Novels, true crime stories, and movies have increasingly portrayed stories that depict the endeavors of forensic scientists in uncovering unsuspected homicides, identifying the guilty parties, and occasionally helping to exculpate certain suspects or exonerate previously convicted people serving life sentences or facing eventual execution for murders that they did not commit.

An Introduction to the Work of a Medical Examiner by John J. Miletich and Tia Laura Lindstrom could not have been published at a more propitious time. The authors have done an excellent job in depicting the professional activities of forensic pathologists. The thoroughly detailed functions of medical examiners (and forensic pathologists serving as or employed by coroners) are presented in an interesting fashion designed to entertain as well as educate the readers of this new book. Forensic science students at all academic levels, practicing physicians and attorneys, *CSI* aficionados, and murder mystery devotees will be delighted with this volume. Learning in a more specific and detailed manner about what goes on in the real world of the forensic pathologist and other forensic scientists by reading this book will undoubtedly serve to increase the knowledge, heighten the awareness, and add to the emotional pleasure of anyone involved with or just plain fascinated by the work performed by modern-day, so-called "medical detectives."

Cyril H. Wecht, M.D., J.D.

ACKNOWLEDGMENTS

FROM JOHN:

Thanks to my co-author, Tia Lindstrom. It was a pleasure to work with her.

I also want to thank the library information desk staff at the Alberta Government Library—7th Street Plaza Site, Concordia University College of Alberta, Edmonton Public Library, Grant MacEwan College, and Northern Alberta Institute of Technology.

I also extend my thanks to the instructors whose general interest courses I attended and who are affiliated with the Office of the Chief Medical Examiner of Alberta, Royal Canadian Mounted Police, and Edmonton Police Service.

I am especially grateful to Debbie Carvalko, Senior Acquisitions Editor, Psychology, Health, and Social Work, at Praeger Publishers, for her commitment to the publication of this book. I very much appreciate her assistance and patience.

FROM TIA:

I'd like to thank Kevin Lindstrom for his patience, smarts, and good humor, as well as my childcare team for their commitment and care: my mother, Ilze; niece, Tia; and brother, Colin. I would also particularly like to thank my co-author John Miletich for inviting me to work on this book. His intelligence and easygoing nature are much appreciated.

I'm grateful to Dr. Cyril Wecht and Dr. Marcella Fierro for their generosity with their time and knowledge. I would also like to thank our editor, Debbie Carvalko, for her help, advice, and kindness.

INTRODUCTION: AN ADVOCATE FOR THE DEAD

YOU MAY HAVE heard the saying "the answers are always in the body," possibly from the mouth of fictional medical examiner Jordan Cavanaugh in the NBC TV series *Crossing Jordan*. Real-life medical examiners have their own mottos, including the Latin words *Mortuí vivós docent*. The dead teach the living. But while every death scene presents medical examiners with clues to a biological mystery, in the real world, answers are not always so clear-cut or readily attained—contrary to most episodes of *CSI: Miami*.

Some side effects of fictional forensic TV programs are described by Orange County Chief Medical Examiner Jan Garavaglia in "Real Life CSI," a December 2005 *Larry King Live* broadcast on CNN. Garavaglia notes, "[t]hey [the audience] do seem to think that there's some type of forensic magic for every case. And I'm in the trenches every day and a lot of our cases just don't have any forensic magic to them . . . but yet they're expecting it."

She adds that she's had family members tell her that cases she's ruled accidental should be investigated as homicides, based on what they've learned from watching *CSI* programs. But while television has perhaps given some audiences an unrealistic view of medical examiner work and forensics in general—DNA analysis, for example, can take weeks if not months to complete, never mind the few days of fictional TV time—it has also given us insight into the working lives of actual medical examiners. Thanks to forensic pathologists such as Michael M. Baden, who hosts *HBO: Autopsy*, as well as Garavaglia, also known for her Discovery Health Channel show, *Dr. G: Medical Examiner*, many TV viewers have developed a deep appreciation for forensic science—and the minds involved in their quest for truth.

For high-profile forensic pathologist Cyril H. Wecht, who has appeared on TV to discuss controversial cases, the job is all about what he can do to benefit public welfare, health, and safety, as well as the justice system. A medical-legal and forensic science consultant, attorney, author, and lecturer (with a list of credentials too long to include here), Wecht has been consulted on Elvis Presley's death, the O.J. Simpson and JonBenet Ramsey cases, and Vincent Foster's death, among many others. Wecht was the coroner and then the medical examiner for Allegheny County, Pennsylvania, until January 2006. He continues his successful private practice in Pittsburgh.

In an interview for this book, Wecht credits his twin interests of medicine and law for drawing him to this field. Although his education gave him a good foundation for the job, he notes that in the early days of his career, some things still caught him a little off guard.

"You're surprised in a sense that even though you do four years of pathology, you don't deal with maggots crawling over a dead body or autoerotic hangings," he explains. Asked what it is like to perform an autopsy, he says it's not something that particularly excites him, but it does make him think:

The first time you do it, it's strange seeing a body cut open—but this happens in medical school, not when you begin work in a medical examiner's office. It makes you think of what is the meaning of life. Everyone philosophizes in different ways, but this is the work we do. A colorectal surgeon looks in people's behinds and a gynecologist looks in women's vaginas. I'm sorry to be crude, but you do what you have to do.

Wecht, who sounds on the phone as though he's closer to age sixty than to his seventy-eight years, pauses and adds, "I think about the meaning of life, especially with deaths of infants and children, and if I see a woman who could have lived if she'd had a tumor removed."

In spite of all the technological advances, Wecht says medical examiners continue to focus on scene investigation and autopsy—done with meticulous attention as their work is often under close courtroom scrutiny: "You still have to deal with the basics and what the body tells you, which hasn't changed in hundreds of years."

And his biggest on-the-job kick? "What gives me a thrill is when I can do something that gives me an answer in a case to show someone's innocent, or that no one's guilty—also on the civil side. And in making a contribution of a scientific nature that aids the justice system."

Those inspired to join this fascinating field will have a long journey ahead—about thirteen to fifteen years of education after high school, including college, medical school, residency, and, in many cases, the completion of a forensic pathology fellowship. A board-certified medical examiner (ME) is a medical doctor, often with specialized training in forensic pathology, a branch of pathology focusing on patients who died sudden, violent, or unexpected deaths. This specialist is an appointed official and is qualified to testify as an expert witness in court.

Some counties in the United States, however, use the old coroner system inherited from England. Coroners are elected officials who may or may not have medical training. The laws of a particular jurisdiction will specify if the coroner needs to be a physician. Often a county's access to adequate funding determines its ability to pay for a medical examiner and the necessary facilities, although rural areas with low rates of violent or unexpected deaths may not need a full-time physician medical examiner. In some counties almost anyone can become a coroner. Although paramedics and sheriffs may be logical choices, it's all up to the electorate.

The word "coroner" is derived from the word "crowner." The crowner's job was to know about deaths during late twelfth-century England, to ensure death duties were paid to King Richard the Lion-Hearted. As a King's representative, the crowner was usually a knight or landowner who investigated suspected homicides and suicides to determine how the dead person's property should be divided. Sometimes days passed before he arrived to inspect the body and preside over jury proceedings.

The medical examiner system was introduced in Massachusetts in 1877, but MEs did not have the right to order autopsies until the 1940s. Nor did those early MEs have a central toxicology lab. The modern medical examiner system began in New York City in 1918, where the first NYC medical examiner was Dr. Charles Norris, professor of pathology at Columbia University and director of Bellevue Hospital laboratories. This system has slowly replaced or combined with the coroner system in many areas.

Besides the obvious advantages of having a knowledgeable doctor examine death scenes (although some coroners hire physicians to do this work), one reason for the new system was to fight political corruption. As medical examiners don't have to please voters, they're more independent of political influence and voter mood. Furthermore, a coroner with limited formal education could not professionally discuss medical or medically related matters with police or other authorities.

Today, the coroner's job depends on the jurisdiction. A non-physician coroner may be required to simply identify the body, notify next of kin, return the deceased's personal items to the family, and complete the death certificate, noting cause and manner of death. He may arrange autopsies. The Los Angeles County Department of Coroner, however, has a Chief Medical Examiner Coroner who is a medical doctor. This department investigates sudden, violent, or unusual deaths in the county. Kentucky goes a step further by combining the coroner/medical examiner systems and giving coroners the authority and powers of peace officers. In places where the coroner is not able to do a necessary autopsy, arrangements are made to bring in a medical examiner.

Regardless of where he practices, the ME's role is to determine cause of death and pronounce some people officially dead: suspected accident victim, suspected suicide, suspected murder victims, or those who died unexpectedly or had unattended deaths. And that is just the beginning. As a forensic death investigator, the medical examiner approaches each case with a fresh mind and some key questions. He learns the health history of the deceased—his patient—as well as the circumstances surrounding the death. He examines the deceased—also referred to as the *decedent*—externally and possibly internally. He also takes advantage of laboratory and other technological and expert resources.

A forensic autopsy can be essential to an investigation. Thorough MEs keep their eyes open for everything—from the obvious to the unexpected—in their search for clues regarding the death. This autopsy helps determine manner of death, specifically one of five ways in which every death is classified: natural, suicide, homicide, accident, or undetermined. Sometimes the manner of death is pending until the ME weighs all the facts and makes a final determination.

Medical examiners may approach a death investigation with six critical questions in mind. Answering them may mean talking to witnesses and authorities, poring over hospital records and police reports, or visiting a death scene.

The first question asks: Who is this (the body)? Learning the deceased's identity is the crux of any investigation. The second question focuses on timing: When did this person get sick, hurt, or die? The third query centers on location: Where did the decedent get hurt or die? Critically injured people can sometimes travel far before they expire; bodies can be moved after death. The fourth question asks for the cause of death: Did the deceased expire from natural causes, from an accident, from violence—or from a combination of factors? The fifth question asks about the manner of death. If this person died from violence, was it suicide, accident, or homicide? The ME must determine the answer in order to write one of the following as manner of death on the death certificate: natural, suicide, accident, homicide, undetermined, or pending investigation. The sixth question stretches outside the boundary of the ME's duties and into the courts: If the deceased was murdered, who did it? The medical examiner can bring forward all the evidence and results from his fact-finding to help provide the answer (Howard n.d.)

In a way, working in forensic science teaches you to think backward. In a November 1986 *Omni Magazine* interview by Douglas Stein, "Thomas Noguchi: Coroner to the Stars," Noguchi, once Chief Medical Examiner-Coroner of Los Angeles County, notes:

> Forensic investigation is like moviemaking but in reverse. We arrive just after the last scene of the cowboy movie—after the cowboys have been surrounded by the American Indians. But did the Union soldiers come to the rescue or not? From the available evidence—fragments of the last scene of the fighting—we try to make each frame, then the one before, and finally the whole movie. We kind of roll the projector backward to the title.

At the beginning of his search for answers to death's questions, whenever possible the ME does a preliminary examination of the dead body at the death scene. This could be where the person died or was critically injured, or where the body was dumped. Key information can be gathered by studying the body in the context of the death scene—evidence that could otherwise be lost to weather conditions, from moving the body, or from other disturbances to the scene. The medical examiner then ensures the decedent is properly transported to the ME's office or morgue, usually in a body bag placed in an unmarked van with tinted windows. The body will likely be kept in a cooler until it is autopsied.

Medical examiners don't autopsy every body referred to their care, of course, nor should they. First, the ME determines if a forensic autopsy is needed by conducting an external examination. This takes place in the autopsy suite at the morgue or ME's office.

As a team player, the ME may involve other specialists, including forensic experts in nursing, entomology, odontology, anthropology, archaeology, and knot analysis. The professional opinions of these experts can influence a medical examiner's final decision in a death investigation.

Much of what happens next in the autopsy suite will be covered in upcoming chapters, but here's a quick run-through. Once the doctor has sufficient cause to continue, he proceeds with a forensic autopsy—an internal examination—after taking necessary photographs and X-rays. He may involve specialists such as forensic entomologists (experts on insects at death scenes).

The medical examiner takes samples from the body to send to labs, possibly for DNA in suspected criminal cases or to identify the decedent, as well as for toxicology. If the body contains a poison not detected by routine toxicological screens, the toxicologist may have to perform more tests—a time-consuming task. Once he feels the picture is complete, the medical examiner fills out the death certificate, a legal document and a public record that includes manner of death. He then releases the body to a funeral home, unless the body is kept as evidence in a legal proceeding such as a murder trial. If this is the case, the ME will likely testify, restricting comments to facts and science. As an expert witness, he is unbiased. His only advocacy is for the dead.

All sorts of people have ended up on the autopsy table in America: from the average Joe and Jane Doe to such famous faces as Michael Jackson, David Carradine, and Anna Nicole Smith. Yet medical examiners investigate relatively few of all deaths reported, as most people die naturally, often from illnesses such as heart disease and cancer. Just to sketch a picture of death in America, during the past few years, approximately 2.4 million people died annually. Of these deaths, approximately 70,000 occurred annually in America's largest city, New York (Ribowsky and Shachtman 2006). In 2003, autopsies were performed on 173,745 bodies—about 7.7 percent of that year's deaths—in 47 states and the District of Columbia, according to the Vital and Health Statistics report, *Autopsy Patterns in 2003*. Autopsies were performed on 14,932 decedents in 2003 in New York State alone, about 9.7 percent of deaths.

Although these numbers include clinical and academic autopsies, the report's authors note that a substantial percentage of deaths fall under the jurisdiction of medical examiners and coroners: those who died under unusual or suspicious circumstances, from violence (accident, suicide, or homicide), unexpectedly, alone, or while not under the treatment of a doctor.

The highest autopsy rates are in the West, the lowest in the South. One standout: the District of Columbia reported autopsies performed in 23.4 percent of deaths there in 2003. Male decedents were more likely to be autopsied, as well as decedents under age 44. Those who died in nursing homes and hospices were the least likely to be autopsied—less than 1 percent in both situations.

Cases are never truly closed, not even after burial. Sometimes an ME reopens a case because new evidence throws doubt on the manner of death initially determined. New technology and advances in DNA typing are making the formerly impossible, possible. Autopsies—and second autopsies—are doable even after a body has been embalmed and/or buried for decades. One example: the notorious Albert DeSalvo, a convict who confessed he was the Boston Strangler, and then later recanted. DeSalvo was buried in 1973, exhumed in 2001, and autopsied, at the request of his family and the family of his last alleged victim. Thanks to DNA technology not available in 1973, New York forensic pathologist Michael Baden and the forensics team came up with some surprising conclusions. This case will be explored further in our chapter on exhumation. While medical examiners must be detail-oriented and meticulous to do their jobs well, they are scientists who sometimes must make judgment calls. Mistakes can be made; others may disagree with findings.

Dr. Wecht caused a stir on September 13, 1979, when he appeared on ABC Television's news program *20/20* to discuss a toxicological report for Elvis Presley, who had died in the bathroom of his home, Graceland, on August 16, 1977. A Memphis medical examiner had told the press that Presley's heart had stopped, probably from cardiovascular disease, and that drugs had played no role in the death. Wecht, who reviewed test results but did not perform an autopsy, came to other, more startling, conclusions: that the King of Rock and Roll had died accidentally from the effect of dangerously combined prescription drugs.

Sometimes it's the family of the deceased who want an autopsy, as did the family of actor David Carradine, a case that will be discussed later in this book. But while unexpected, mysterious celebrity deaths such as Michael Jackson's and Carradine's generate interest worldwide, media investigations and conspiracy theorists have also done their bit to push some medical examiners' cases into the limelight. Consider the deaths of actress Marilyn Monroe, billionaire Robert Maxwell, and White House Counsel Vincent W. Foster, Jr., which also will be discussed later in these pages. Their tragic ends have moved many to ask whether their deaths were suicide or murder.

Amid all of this, the medical examiner remains a spokesperson for the decedent. The role he plays in medical and legal matters makes him a valuable member of society.

By the time the reader reads the first case profile, near the end of this book, the reader will have read a comprehensive overview about the work of medical examiners, the forensic professionals whom medical examiners consult, as well as police criminal investigation experts.

And there are plenty of places to learn more about it. High schools, colleges, and universities in the U.S., Canada, and other countries offer specific courses and programs about death scene investigation. Those who have a passing or layman's interest in death scene investigation may find basic courses in their communities.

It's an exciting field, as the science continues to expand and offer fresh breakthroughs; what may not be known or answerable today could be solved tomorrow.

Meanwhile, for a medical examiner, no murder is too brutal, no suicide too puzzling, no accident too horrific, and no natural disaster too massive to ignore or overlook. *An Introduction to the Work of a Medical Examiner: From Death Scene to Autopsy Suite* places the reader at the scene, indoors or outdoors, regardless of day, time, or season.

1

——•••——

EXPERTS IN DEATH

IT'S ALWAYS WISE to get an expert opinion. So, in considering what it's like to work as a medical examiner, we turned to Dr. Marcella Fierro, the former chief medical examiner of Virginia. One immediate conclusion can be drawn: medical examiner work is not for wimps.

When asked about her job, the forensic pathologist can tell workday stories that make your hair stand on end—and tug at your heart. It's reality without the TV, and it can be harsh.

"In forensics we see a lot of violent deaths, a lot of tragic deaths, a lot of preventable deaths," Fierro explains. "It's someone who goes out to buy a loaf of bread and gets into an accident. It's not expected, they never get to say good-bye. For the family, it's catastrophic. And when a young person dies, all those years are lost."

Fierro, who was the inspiration for Patricia Cornwell's bestselling Kay Scarpetta novels, says some of the worst cases are those that frighten the entire community, such as serial killers and snipers. In one case she describes from 2002, a sniper hid in the trunk of a car and, as his partner drove the vehicle down the road, shot through the hole left from the removed lock.

"Who is going to see some little hole in a trunk with a shooter hiding in there? It scared the socks off people," Fierro says. "What kind of person decides to shoot some poor guy pumping gas, or some woman coming out of the store with her shopping? Also, the people gloated—the shooters—saying [in phone calls to police]: 'You're going to be next, or your children.'"

The doctor also worked on the Virginia Tech massacre and Richmond's Southside Strangler killings. She says the sooner the ME can work with the police to help solve the crimes, the better for the community. Other memorable medical examiner cases are the "sneaky homicides," when someone thinks he or she can get away with murder.

"Some of the sneakiest ones are when somebody kills someone then burns the place down, thinking we won't be able to sort it all out. But we do," says

Fierro. "In places where there's a competent medical examiner system, these cases don't fly by us. Other places without a medical examiner system, they can slip by. But they don't slip by forensic pathologists."

While the job can be hard emotionally for an ME, Fierro says the way to deal with that is to look at what you can do: "We're in a position to see a lot of tragedy but also to do something about it. And that's a very good feeling." Medical examiners can go to court on behalf of the decedent and fight for justice. Or they may discover that a person died from a contagious disease and work to keep the community safe. MEs can also identify other health risks in the community and find ways to inform people.

Fierro recalls a newspaper interview she gave a few years ago after several local people died in fires. During the interview, she recommended the public buy smoke alarms and learn more about fire prevention. "Later I got a call [from the fire department]: the city was sold out of smoke detectors. The statistics that year went from 20 deaths [due to fire] to 5 deaths. Yes, it's sad to see fire deaths, but you can do something about it. I felt like we saved 15 deaths that year, and it [the benefit] carries over. And that's something to be proud of."

Fierro notes that "[w]hen people die of natural disease, it's the end point of a natural process; it's usually not preventable and follows treatment. [In forensics] you see a lot of deaths that are preventable. That's why a forensic pathologist is also a health officer—a lot of what we do is around prevention."

She says good traits for a medical examiner are an innate curiosity, the perseverance to answer a question, and a commitment to truth in terms of criminal justice and public health. Medical examiners must also be prepared to visit some odd sites. In Fierro's experience, these have included burned-out buildings, snake-infested swamps, and train yards.

The part Fierro liked least about her job as medical examiner was waiting for lab results, which could take weeks. Not only did that hold up her cases, but the family would have to wait, too. Her biggest thrill? She says it's when a case came in as one thing but she discovered it was something else: "When I figured out something that nobody knew, now that [was] great."

Fierro, who retired in 2007 after more than thirty years in medical examiner offices, continues to teach at Virginia Institute of Forensic Science and Medicine, as well as do private work, consult for the FBI, and sit on federal panels.

Any science employed in the service of the law is forensic science. Its purpose is to support the unbiased truth. This opens up a wide variety of careers in forensics, including criminalists, engineers, anthropologists, entomologists, biologists, pathologists, toxicologists, psychiatrists, and even artists—such as Donna Cline, a forensic artist who does research, storyboard art, and biomedical illustration for the FOX TV program *Bones*. The medical examiner's role in this search for truth is to investigate the deaths of people who die suddenly, unexpectedly, or violently within her particular jurisdiction, in one of more than 2,000 death investigation jurisdictions in the United States and Canada.

Other criteria that make a death fall within a medical examiner's territory include emergency-room deaths not due to trauma, deaths while in the custody of police or jail, or deaths that occur on the job. Although some coroners may be elected officials with no medical background, an ME has the medical expertise to evaluate the medical history and physical condition of a dead person. As a physician, the ME may practice any branch of medicine and is not always required to be a specialist in death investigation or pathology (Cataldie 2006; National Association of Medical Examiners 2004; Timmermans 2006).

The doctor's specialty does have an impact on her activities as a medical examiner, however. Medical examiners who perform autopsies in death investigations are usually forensic pathologists. This is a specialized area of pathology. Board-certified forensic pathologists have been certified by the American Board of Pathology and have had forensic pathology training or experience. They are also licensed in one or more states. Their duties include performing autopsies to uncover injury, disease, and poisoning in situations that fall within the local medical examiner's or coroner's jurisdiction. They collect medical evidence, including secretions, to document sexual assault as well as to help learn what caused the injuries.

In addition to their medical training, forensic pathologists who work as medical examiners must also have a working knowledge of other areas of science, including DNA technology, toxicology, wound ballistics, trace evidence, and forensic serology. When working as death investigators, these doctors can help assess the death scene as well as how well witness statements match injuries. They assess the collected forensic evidence and determine cause and manner of death. They may be called upon to be expert witnesses and testify about autopsy findings in court. A forensic pathologist is also an expert in the study of causes, development, progression, and consequences of diseases (Death 2004). As an aside, some clinical forensic pathologists investigate sexual assault and child abuse cases with living victims. In these situations, they examine the person for injuries and other evidence, usually on behalf of law enforcement agencies.

Pathologists, meanwhile, are doctors who specialize in natural diseases and who work in private clinics, morgues, labs, or hospitals. They may do autopsies in hospitals or morgues on people who died natural deaths—but not usually to determine cause of death or manner of death in death investigations. In ME offices where the medical examiners don't have a background in forensic pathology—and this is likely in small jurisdictions in the U.S.—an ME with the relevant background is brought in from another jurisdiction to perform the autopsy.

Forensic pathology is a small specialty. In spite of the popularity of forensic investigation television shows, forensic medical programs aren't packing in the students. Only about thirty to forty med students per year complete the training and sit for the exams to be board-certified. Although there are about 800,000 medical doctors in the U.S., only a fraction of them are board-certified, full-time forensic pathologists. Numbers for 2003 show 989 board-certified forensic pathologists, with only about 600 of them active practitioners and fewer than 400 working full-time (NAME 2004). In fact, since 1959, when the exam was first offered to board-certify forensic pathologists, only about 1,300 doctors have chosen this career path. Most young doctors may prefer to help patients who are alive or may wish to avoid any chance of working with rotting, slimy, insect-infested bodies. It also takes at least nine years of formal education after college to become a forensic pathologist, including med school, and, ironically, the pay may be much less of what could be earned in pathology or by physicians in general. It may be hard to persuade a young doctor to pursue forensic pathology and accept less pay when she's in debt for her expensive medical school education.

Yet these specialists are essential to an effective justice system. Their skills can uncover previously unsuspected homicides as well as deaths that may alert the forensic pathologist to a public health risk. These highly trained medical examiners can also benefit victims of crime by helping to catch perpetrators.

A case in Canada illustrates the dangers of having too small a pool of forensic pathologists—especially well-trained forensic pathologists. Dr. Charles Smith, seen as a leading Canadian expert in pediatric forensic pathology in the 1990s, was found to have little real forensic expertise after his errors led to several wrongful prosecutions—including Bill Mullins-Johnson, who was convicted of raping and murdering his four-year-old niece and spent twelve years in prison. Later, expert pathologists found no forensic evidence of sexual assault or violence, and determined the little girl died a natural death. Mullins-Johnson was released on bail in 2005 and acquitted in 2007. Smith's status in the field was due almost entirely to the fact that there was no one else with the training or experience to check him. This case sparked the creation of Canada's first forensic pathology residency program at the University of Toronto in 2009.

A shortage of forensic pathologists means some practitioners may be exceeding the recommended caseloads just to keep up with demand, and thus risking mistakes and burnout. Pathologist practitioners who don't have forensic training may also be doing medicolegal autopsies, or autopsies performed to answer questions about identity, cause of death, and circumstances of death that may help police solve crimes. Families in some areas may wait months to have the question of their loved one's death resolved—if ever—as well as any lawsuits or insurance claims settled. And while there is a decline in hospital autopsies, the need for medicolegal autopsies increases with the population. Some estimates suggest that 800 to 1,000 full-time forensic pathologists are needed to adequately serve all areas of the U.S.

Physician medical examiners who wish to be more proficient in death investigation, however, can take specialized training, such as that offered through the National Association of Medical Examiners (NAME). Established in 1966, NAME is the national professional organization for medical examiners who perform medicolegal death investigations of interest to the American public. In addition to supporting the professional development of physician death investigators, the organization disseminates professional information to help improve death investigation in America and other countries. Membership is open to all physicians, investigators, and administrators who are active in medicolegal death investigation. The organization has close to 1,000 members, about half of whom are forensic pathologists (not all American forensic pathologists or medical examiners are members, however).

Another organization of interest here is the American Academy of Forensic Sciences (AAFS), a professional society established in 1948 that promotes the advancement of the forensic sciences. AAFS has nearly 6,000 members in a wide variety of disciplines.

One of the medical examiner's key forensic tools for uncovering the truth of what killed the decedent is, of course, the autopsy. An autopsy is a detailed, surgically invasive medical examination of a person's body after death to help determine the cause of death. The word *autopsy* is derived from the Greek word *autopsia*, which means "seeing for oneself." It is an opportunity for observation. An autopsy conducted by a medical examiner differs from a hospital autopsy, in that an autopsy ordered by an ME or coroner is done so with the authority of the law and with the purpose of determining cause of death and solving other death investigation questions. The ME does not require permission from next of kin, who has no say over the autopsy. In this case, a complete autopsy is almost always done, meaning that all body cavities and organs, as well as the head, are examined in the search for clues.

A hospital autopsy, however, is usually performed on people whose cause of death is known. In this case, the purpose is more academic: to determine the development of the disease as well as effects of treatment, and to locate any undiagnosed illness that contributed to the death. The deceased's next of kin must give permission and may limit the procedure to certain areas of the body. For example, the decedent's head may be excluded in a limited autopsy, while only specific organs are examined in a selective autopsy.

Cause of death is a key term for a medical examiner. It means something that killed a person, such as a knife thrust into a person's heart (Baden and Roach 2001). The cause of death is a condition, a syndrome, or what first directly created the specific wound or injury. Death happens when a person's physiology and biochemistry alter in a way that is incompatible with life. Violence or disease can lead to states that lead to death. For example, hypoxia, or oxygen deficiency, is incompatible with life and can be caused by advanced arteriosclerotic, coronary heart disease. It can also be caused by strangulation. It's up to the medical examiner to find the correct cause of death: strangulation or coronary heart disease. Hypoxia would be the mechanism of death in either case. Instead of a single cause of death, the medical examiner may find a variety of contributors to the death: one or several natural diseases; a single injury or multiple wounds; a solitary syndrome or a number of syndromes. Details from the deceased patient's death scene, autopsy, toxicology tests, and X-rays, as well as his or her medical history, must all be weighed to determine cause of death (Cause 2004; Death 2005).

The term *manner of death* refers to the way the person died: accident, suicide, homicide, natural, or undetermined. "Pending" can substitute for the manner of death on a death certificate until a final determination is made (Baden and Roach 2001).

A medical examiner or death investigator usually becomes involved in a case after receiving a call from a detective at a death scene. In some cases, a death investigator performs duties similar to those of a medical examiner, but may lack the advanced medical and legal education of an ME. The death investigator may have forensic nursing or criminal justice expertise and will go to the death scene as the medical examiner's representative. Forensic pathologists, however, are sometimes referred to as "death investigators." Death investigators are called upon because medical examiners and a few associate medical examiners in high-caseload jurisdictions cannot always respond to every death scene. In these busy jurisdictions, the ME and associate medical examiners get their information about specific cases from police, hospital, and other reports. They focus more on autopsies than on scene investigations.

But the renowned and at times controversial former Los Angeles County Chief Medical Examiner-Coroner, Dr. Thomas T. Noguchi, made it a point to attend death scenes whenever possible, in spite of his high-caseload jurisdiction. Noguchi attended the death scenes of and performed autopsies on many public figures, including Robert F. Kennedy in 1968 and Marilyn Monroe in 1962. The popular fictional TV series *Quincy*, starring Jack Klugman, was based on Noguchi, who was often referred to in the media as the "Coroner to the Stars."

Here is an example of how a call plays out at the medical examiner's office, beginning with a hypothetical outdoor death scene. A police detective calls the ME's office and relates all the relevant immediate facts: the body is an adult male, and three apparently unopened glassine envelopes containing a white substance were found near the body. The death investigator (DI) speaking to the detective confirms that the death is reportable, as it falls within the jurisdiction of the medical examiner. Reportable deaths in most jurisdictions are suspicious, sudden, unexpected, unexplained, traumatic, or medically unattended. A medically unattended death is defined as occurring outside a hospital or long-term care facility and outside of the care of a physician—or any recent medical examinations.

Typically, two death investigators and a forensic scene photographer respond to reportable deaths. Depending on the death scene, the team might also include a criminalist, an expert who recognizes, collects, documents, analyzes, and preserves physical evidence, including firearms, blood, drugs, and fibers. The team greets a police officer, whose duties include identifying every person at the scene. Team members write down their names, agency/affiliation, and the time they arrived on a sign-in sheet. They note the police incident number for their records. Later at the medical examiner's office, they can use this number to access information about a specific incident more quickly on the computer than by typing in the decedent's name or death scene address.

First responders and the detective on the scene brief the death investigators about the decedent and death scene. They may speculate about the cause, mechanism, and manner of death. The team then dons latex gloves and crosses the "Police Line—Do-Not-Cross" barrier, being careful not to contaminate potential evidence the police have pointed out: the glassine envelopes. The scene forensic photographer takes pictures of the deceased from a variety of angles and also photographs the surrounding area so the body can be seen within the context of nearby trees and a wire-mesh fence. The soil around the body is dry and hard; the death investigators search unsuccessfully for any footprints to photograph. They note the position of the body, looking for clues to indicate whether the decedent fell to the ground and died where a jogger found him earlier; the body was dumped or thrown from a vehicle; or the body was dragged, leaving a trail of blood, leaves, or dirt. They see no fresh tire tracks. The death investigators look for obvious trauma on the decedent, but do not see any. They look for indications that insects have colonized the body, but find none. The life cycles of insects such as flies and beetles are useful to death scene investigations, as these bugs can help determine time of death.

One death investigator easily flexes the decedent's fingers, showing the body is not in full rigor mortis (a postmortem stiffness that develops gradually and lasts about seventy-two hours). The DI concludes the decedent has probably been dead for several hours. A body in full rigor mortis is so stiff it is virtually impossible to manipulate any part of it. An attempt to bend the body could break its bones. In fact, a flat body in full rigor mortis could be placed across the tops of two chairs like a plank. It would remain in that position until it lost full rigor.

The glassine envelopes, meanwhile, suggest the decedent could be a drug dealer or drug user. The death investigators look unsuccessfully for readily visible injection sites on the skin, such as the forearms—areas easily accessible without completely undressing the body. If the sites exist, the medical examiner will likely find them when she examines the unclothed body. She may do her inspection with a magnifying glass.

While searching the body, the death investigators take great care to avoid getting punctured by anything sharp, particularly a syringe that could infect them with AIDS, hepatitis, and other serious diseases. One approach is to tap pockets with a pen or pencil and listen for the sound of a hard object, like a syringe. Warily, they probe the decedent's pockets for personal effects: wallet, credit cards, a Social Security card, keys, and any other items that may offer clues to the person's identity or why he died. They find no syringes among the personal effects. A DI positively identifies the decedent by comparing his face with the photograph and other information on his driver's license.

As an aside, sometimes a jogger found dead in a park or elsewhere has no identification on his body, but may have his car key in his pocket or wear it dangling from a chain around his neck. Later in the day, detectives may try out this key on cars left in the park or neighborhood. Once they find the car that matches the key, the investigators search the car for any relevant information and run the license tag number through the Department of Motor Vehicles computer.

In our example, the decedent's name matches a moniker given to police by a small group of onlookers when police first arrived on the scene and asked if any knew the dead person. A DI collects the glassine envelopes to initiate *chain of custody*, a procedure to protect and document the movement of evidence from its initial collection site to its entry as evidence in court. This procedure includes the name and agency or affiliation of every person who handled the evidence; the date and time the evidence was collected or transferred; and the reason the evidence was transferred.

The death investigators place the body on a clean sheet and cover the decedent's hands with paper bags, taping them at the forearms or securing the bags with elastic bands. This preserves potential trace evidence: hair, fibers, or a tiny piece of skin that may have lodged under the decedent's fingernails if he, even momentarily, struggled with a perpetrator before dying. Genetic material—or DNA—from a sample of skin caught under a fingernail could be used to identify a perpetrator. Paper bags are preferred over plastic bags when attempting to preserve trace evidence as condensation may form in plastic bags and degrade evidence, including blood and gunshot residue.

In our hypothetical case, the death investigators have finished attaching paper bags to the decedent's hands. A DI presses the sharp end of a probe thermometer into the side of the body to record the liver temperature. Although inserting the thermometer penetrates the deceased's skin and pierces the liver, this is not a problem forensically as the DI records that the thermometer produced this injury. He also records the ambient temperature, the temperature of the air around the body—this measurement will vary according to the distance from the body it's taken.

The death investigators lift the deceased into a body bag that they label, lock, and then slide into the back of an unmarked medical examiner's van. They remove their latex gloves, place them in a biohazard receptacle in the back of the van, and wash their hands with a liquid antibacterial soap. Next, they interview witnesses, including the jogger who found the body and the onlooker who told police he knows the name of the man lying on the ground. They will also talk to the decedent's family members. Police will sometimes discretely photograph onlookers at the death scene. They know the killer or a key material witness may be among the onlookers at some suspicious death or obvious homicide scenes.

The death investigators receive the investigation reports from the police and keep the medical examiner informed about the investigation. They can see no apparent reason for the death: it appears the decedent literally dropped dead. But the ME will make the final determination regarding cause, mechanism, and manner of death, likely after an autopsy—something the death investigators will recommend. If this becomes a homicide investigation, the DI team will have additional duties that include preparing subpoenas for witnesses and testifying in court. At last, the team members sign out and leave for the medical examiner's office.

Emotions can run high at a death scene investigation, especially when the decedent's family or friends are present. Reactions to death vary with the individual. Some may be passive and sullen; others may be loud and aggressive. Family or friends may be consumed with grief and police may have to restrain them. Manic individuals may attack police who initially informed them about the death. A person who may appear to be no threat may suddenly become enraged. The lives of paramedics and the medical examiner may be in danger (Noguchi and Di Mona 1983; Ramsland 2001; Wecht 2004).

Dealing with strangers in general can be dangerous. On Christmas morning 1994 in Philadelphia, two paramedics on their way to a maternity call were flagged down by a man in distress. They stopped their vehicle to help him and another man lying in the road, but the second man got up and leapt at them with a knife, according to a *New York Times* article, "Man Attacks Paramedics Who Offered Aid," published Monday, December 26. The paramedics treated their own minor injuries before returning to work. The pregnant woman, meanwhile, told other emergency workers she would go to the hospital by car.

This kind of trouble is one reason why Louisiana law gives medical examiners the authority of a peace officer, including the right to carry a firearm. Louisiana State Medical Examiner and author Louis Cataldie often brings his .32 Kel-Tec semiautomatic pistol to death scenes. Cataldie's wife, DeAnn Cataldie, a psychiatric nurse and registered medicolegal death investigator, carries a .357 Smith & Wesson when she works cases (Cataldie 2006; Miletich 2003).

Police officers, paramedics, emergency medical technicians, and firefighters respond daily to calls for help. Sometimes people die by the time help arrives. Typically, the first responder looks for visible injuries on the person and then checks for a carotid pulse. The carotid pulse can be detected by gently palpating one of the two carotid arteries found on either side of the neck below the jawbone. These arteries carry blood from the heart to the brain. As one responder performs this check, another responder cuts away clothing from the person's chest and then applies electrocardiogram patches to test for electrical activity in the chest. A flat line appears on the monitor when the heart has stopped. If the person is not breathing and has no pulse, the first responders check for rigor mortis (postmortem stiffening) as well as livor mortis, a settling of blood in parts of the body closest to the ground. This produces a purplish red discoloration of the skin. When a body shows these conditions, the person can be declared dead (Wecht 2004).

In some cases, a whole body is not available to declare dead. In late December 1978, Cook County Medical Examiner Dr. Robert Stein found himself on his knees at 8213 Summerdale Avenue in Norwood Park, a suburb of Chicago, Illinois. This was serial killer John Wayne Gacy's house. Along with investigators, Stein had put on a disposable paper jumpsuit and made his way into the dark, 28- by 38-foot crawlspace under the 1950s home. As medical examiner, Stein's specific duties here were to view the remains, determine if they were human, pronounce any remains or bodies dead, and assign a morgue identification number to those bodies or remains. Police were there to remove the remains as well as any articles of clothing found nearby.

An investigator showed Stein a small object that he identified as a human kneecap. The medical examiner's work was just beginning. Later, an unearthed body began to bloat rapidly from a buildup of methane and hydrogen sulfide. Stein had to cut open the corpse's abdomen to release the pressure. Investigators took care to place each body or set of remains in its own body bag, put each bag in a separate wire litter, and carry them to the waiting morgue van. At the end of each day's work, Stein and one or more senior police officers updated the press at the crime scene. By New Year's Eve, the body count was twenty-seven.

In what appeared to be another gruesome discovery, investigators found frozen meat and a container of a bloodlike substance in Gacy's garage. Stein had the meat and contents of the container analyzed. Test results showed the meat was not human flesh; the container's liquid contents were stewed tomatoes.

Investigators used missing person information, dental records, X-rays, fingerprints, and personal effects including jewelry and keys to identify victims. In 1980, Gacy was convicted of murdering thirty-three young men, whom he had strangled to death. Fourteen years later, the fifty-two-year-old Gacy was executed by lethal injection (Sullivan and Maiken 1983).

Not all decedents are so obviously the victims of murder, but medical examiners cannot uncover crimes if suspicious or unexpected deaths are not reported. In a series of articles in 2000 and 2001, the *Charlotte Observer* revealed that as many as 2,500 cases of unnatural death statewide in North Carolina were not reported between 1993 and 1998. One reason noted was that some doctors didn't report deaths when they thought the deaths did not result from a crime. These doctors may not have known that assault victim deaths are reportable even when the victims die months after the assault. A number of doctors acknowledged they did not report certain deaths because county medical examiners had inconsistent policies. And when these North Carolina doctors called in reportable deaths, at times medical examiners did not hear about them because of bureaucratic errors due to staff shortages, inadequately trained staff, or limited resources. Families of people who died in that state may never know what killed their loved ones.

Mistakes can also be made if the ME doesn't take full advantage of his toolkit, particularly the autopsy option. In the following case in Moore County, North Carolina, an autopsy led to a correction in a cause-of-death decision.

Shortly after midnight on July 6, 1996, thirty-nine-year-old Gary Blyther and his girlfriend, Rebecca Ann DeLouise, broke into the house of Blyther's grandmother, Hattie Blyther, age eighty-five. Gary Blyther, high on crack cocaine, smothered his grandmother with a pillow and stole the Social Security money she had hidden in her bra. When police discovered Hattie Blyther's body in bed, her bra was torn and her money was gone.

Yet a Moore County medical examiner visited the death scene and concluded that heart disease was the cause of death. That ruling didn't sit well with Moore County Sheriff's Deputy James Carpenter. Hattie Blyther's doctor had told the deputy that, although the grandmother had heart disease, he was surprised she died from it. Later, when deputies in another county questioned Gary Blyther about an unrelated offense, Blyther thought they knew about the murder and talked about it. The case was reopened. Hattie Blyther's body was exhumed and then autopsied by North Carolina Chief Medical Examiner Dr. John Butts, who found no signs of a recent heart attack. He changed the cause of death to homicide by suffocation. Gary Blyther was convicted of first-degree murder in 1998 and received a sentence of life in prison. His girlfriend was convicted of conspiracy to commit murder and received a sentence of up to ten years.

The Blyther case illustrates how medical examiners use different standards, leading to different results. In the *Charlotte Observer* articles, Dr. Butts reportedly agreed that local medical examiners had different standards. He noted that he had little control over the more than 530 doctors who served as part-time death investigators.

Cause of death can be difficult to determine accurately if a doctor doesn't consider the deceased patient's medical history. The following North Carolina case illustrates how an autopsy revealed a death was due to an event that happened weeks before, thanks to the persistence of the decedent's family members.

In Pitt County in 1996, seventy-six-year-old Harvey Newton was in a car accident. Less than a month later, he died. The doctor who saw his body decided that Newton died of natural causes, so the medical examiner was not notified. Newton's relatives, however, were concerned about an insurance policy and suspected that the car accident had caused the senior's death. They contacted the medical examiner, who had the body exhumed and autopsied. The autopsy showed that a blood clot in Newton's fractured leg traveled to his lungs and caused his death. Accident, therefore, replaced natural as the manner of death.

Medical examiners and death investigators are human, and thus mistakes will likely be made from time to time. Even so, improvements are in the works for North Carolina's quality of death investigations. In 2001, a task force created by the Department of Health and Human Services concluded that North Carolina should establish five regional centers staffed by trained investigators and forensic pathologists, who would support local medical examiners. North Carolina actually began the process decades ago by establishing a statewide medical examiner system in the late 1960s. The system eliminated the need for coroners and relied on appointed doctors to conduct death investigations. Dr. Page Hudson, who created the system, planned to open regional offices staffed by forensic pathologists, but the system was not successful statewide. He retired as chief medical examiner in 1986 (Cenziper February 12, 2001; Cenziper February 14, 2001; Cenziper November/December 2001; Cenziper December 30, 2001; Cenziper, Garloch, and Mellnik February 12, 2001).

Other states have solved reporting problems with doctor education and improved death certificate tracking, as well as specific reporting guidelines. New Mexico, for example, relies on doctors and lay investigators trained in death investigation. Forensic pathologists conduct every ME autopsy in the state at a single center. In Virginia, forensic pathologists perform autopsies in regional centers alongside police crime labs and university medical centers. After all, forensic work is team oriented. Sharing information and developing strong networks among forensic professionals enhances the environment for effective death investigations—and, ultimately, answering the key critical questions of what happened to each life, case-by-case.

To that end, the medical examiner's approach was already summed up more than a hundred years ago by the nineteenth-century French medico-legalist Dr. P.C.H. Brouardel: "If the law has made you a witness, remain a man of science. You have no victim to avenge, no guilty or innocent person to convict or save—you must bear testimony within the limits of science."

2

<hr>

DEATH AND THE HUMAN BODY

TELEVISION IS LITTERED with corpses. From crime dramas and thrillers to news documentaries and true-life forensic investigation programs, corporal gore and decay are not hard to find. The viewing public's tolerance—and in some cases their taste—for graphic detail has grown with the development of the small screen.

Most members of the TV audience, kids included, see more dead bodies in one week of regular programming than they will ever see in person. But contrary to what many of these viewers may think, death is not one specific moment. It is a process.

To an observer, a natural death can appear to creep up quietly. First, breathing stops. Stillness settles over the body. The person's jaw muscles relax. Depending on his body position, dentures, if worn, may fall out of his mouth. The body may slump or sag. His face becomes pale and drawn.

It's commonly thought that when people die, their bladders and bowels will empty. Pelvic muscles and the smooth muscle in the rectum may relax after death, but defecation doesn't automatically occur. This is because these muscles must contract for defecation to happen. However, if a body is moved, a relaxed anal sphincter may release fecal matter at the end of the rectum (Ribowsky and Shachtman 2006).

A human body needs specific conditions to continue living, including fresh supplies of oxygen for the brain and nourished blood to flow through the veins. The brain is greedy, requiring more than 25 percent of the oxygen a person inhales. This leaves little leeway for major disruptions, such as a heart attack or gunshot wounds that prevent vital organs from functioning.

During the death process, the brain dies first because its cells are more sensitive to the lack of oxygen and glucose supply than any other organ. When a person stops breathing, the brain starts to lose brain cells within minutes. Unlike other body tissues, the neurons of the human central nervous system have almost no ability to regenerate after an injury. The brain can survive only for about six minutes after the heart stops. The person rapidly loses consciousness, becomes comatose, and then brain death occurs (Baden 2006). A person is considered brain-dead when his brain and brain stem are permanently and irreversibly damaged; he is past the point of no return. The brain stem, the lowest part of the brain, connects to the spinal cord; the upper regions of the brain exchange information with the spinal cord and peripheral nerves. The brain stem oversees breathing, blood pressure, and heart rate. Without these essential components of the central nervous system, consciousness and functionality end.

One view of this is that the brain-dead body is simply a network of living cells. But some controversy over this lingers, as some brain-dead patients can absorb nutrients, fight infections, heal wounds, and carry out a pregnancy (Mori, Shingu, and Nakao 2009). Cerebral death, also known as the "persistent vegetative state," means the end of activity in the cerebral cortices and is not alone considered brain death, as the permanence of cerebral dysfunction is not easily predicted and can be misdiagnosed. Also, in this state, brain stem functions that control respiratory centers, the autonomic nervous system, endocrine system, and immune system may be functioning. Cerebral death means a cessation of consciousness—but systems vital for preserving life may continue for months or years (Mathers and Frankel 2007; Mori, Shingu, and Nakao 2009).

In most states, legal death is brain death; this means that a legal declaration of death is not dependent on the cessation of heartbeat or blood circulation. To determine brain death, there must be a recognized cause of coma, something that will explain the irreversible end of brain function. Although brain death means all functions of the central nervous system—cortex and brain stem—are inactive, some spinal cord-related and muscle reflexes may continue to function (Mathers and Frankel 2007). Factors that determine brain death are irreversible unconsciousness; irreversible lack of brain stem reflexes; and the absence of anything that may have depressed or impaired the person's central nervous system function, such as drugs or hypothermia. The patient is in a deep coma (Mathers and Frankel 2007; Mori, Shingu, and Nakao 2009).

The Model Brain Death Act of 1979 states that a person is dead when either of two conditions is met: the person's body has permanently lost its ability to function regarding circulation and respiration, or the person's brain, including the brain stem, has irreversibly ceased functioning (Puswella, DeVita, and Arnold 2005). However, other organs can continue to "live" on a cellular level after the brain—and, therefore, the person—has died. This makes organ donation possible.

A brain-dead person's body can be kept alive with a ventilator and life-supporting medications. As long as the body is connected to a ventilator and its body temperature, blood pressure, pulse remain consistent, fluid and nutrition needs are met, the skin is warm, the chest rises and falls as breathing continues, and tepid urine flows through tubing draining the bladder, the body is alive. Once disconnected from life support, a brain-dead person's body is no longer alive, not even artificially (Chen 2005).

The heart tends to be the last organ to cease functioning. It can beat for fifteen to twenty minutes without oxygen after the brain has died, according to *HBO: Autopsy* star Dr. Michael Baden (Ask n.d.). This is because the heart's muscle tissue can temporarily get energy from within the body even when oxygen has been virtually depleted. About twenty minutes after the heart has stopped, most organs will cease functioning. Corneas can stay viable for twenty-four hours, while tendons, bones, and muscles can be used for donation for a couple of days. If a lung or liver is to be transplanted after the brain is dead, the organ must be kept alive with oxygen, electrolytes, and fluids—usually in a medical facility where the transplant will be performed (Baden 2006).

Several processes happen after death that can offer medical examiners valuable clues in a death investigation. One of these is temperature, the first key sign of death. Cooling, or *algor mortis*, is also referred to as "the chill of death." Generally speaking, body temperature after death remains relatively level for thirty minutes to five hours and then drops at a constant rate. In theory, the rate of cooling drops rapidly as the temperature of the body approaches the temperature of its environment. But this may not be true if the person's body temperature was not normal at death. Other factors may affect body cooling. The greater the surface area of the body relative to its mass—such as in a slim person—the faster it will cool; the more obese the body, the slower the heat loss. Clothing insulates the body and decreases cooling, while cooling is more rapid in a humid atmosphere than in a dry atmosphere, as moist air is a better conductor of heat.

While affected by many factors, the decedent's body temperature is still an important measurement for medical examiners, especially at a death scene. This way the body's temperature can be compared to the ambient temperature, to help the ME determine how long the body has been at the death scene. The ME typically uses a ten- to twelve-inch-long thermometer with a digital display and range of 0 degrees to 50 degrees Centigrade. If there is no reason to suspect sexual assault, he inserts the thermometer into the rectum or through the abdomen and into the liver. He makes small slits in the clothing to expose the rectum if the clothing cannot be pushed to one side. An alternative is to shift or cut clothing, make a puncture in the abdomen, and then insert the thermometer.

Another way to estimate a time of death is by measuring potassium levels in vitreous humor (a clear, colorless gel in the posterior part of the eyeball). This is because although the body's cells begin to break down and release potassium into the bloodstream about an hour or two following death, this process happens at a slower and much more predictable rate in vitreous humor. Also, temperature does not affect this process. To check potassium levels, the medical examiner inserts a very fine needle into the eyeball to withdraw the humor. She is careful not to touch the eyeball (she may do this test as part of the external exam at the ME's office). Medical examiners use formulas for potassium levels to establish an approximate time of death, usually to within a couple of hours. However, this test does not reveal useful information if used on a person who has been dead more than twelve hours (Wecht, Saitz, and Curriden 2003).

While it's an important step in an investigation, medical examiners acknowledge the data used to determine time of death has its limitations. On TV or in a book, an ME may say John Doe died at 7:15 P.M., but real-world medical examiners may give a time in a range of several hours; too many variables affect accuracy. In court, a lawyer can use these variables to strengthen any doubts a jury may have about the ME's credibility (Temple 2005).

The next key sign of death is *livor mortis*. About half an hour to two hours after death, this typically purplish discoloration appears on the skin on the lowest parts of the body in respect to the ground. Also known as hypostasis, postmortem lividity, or the "bruising of death," livor mortis is the result of gravity's pull on red blood cells that are no longer actively circulating, making them sink to the lowest vessels.

When pressure is applied to areas with livor mortis, they blanch, or turn white. Later, red blood cells break down (hemolyze) and the hemoglobin—the iron-containing pigment in these cells—leaches out of the blood vessels into surrounding muscle tissues. Pressure can then no longer create this blanching effect, as the hemoglobin has become "fixed." Like temperature, livor is not a reliable variable for accurately determining time of death because it does not become fixed over a specific time period.

The qualities of the deceased person's livor mortis can offer information helpful to a death investigation, however. A person who dies while lying on his back, and is not moved until the livor is fixed, will show the purplish bruising only on his back. Patches of livor on different areas of the body indicate the body was moved before livor became fixed. Livor does not fade away. One note: Livor mortis is not always purple; sometimes it will be red or pink. The blood of a person who died of carbon monoxide poisoning will continue to be bright red after death; the blood of someone who died of cyanide poisoning will be pink (Anatomic 2004; Green 2000; Owen 2000; Ramsland 2001).

If you've ever wondered why a corpse is called a "stiff" in slang, this is why: *rigor mortis*. Rigor is a progressive stiffening of a dead person's muscles that usually begins in an hour or two and is complete in four to six hours, depending on the body's ambient temperature, body fat, amount of muscle mass, and any physical activity before death. As a general rule, the rigor comes within twelve hours, lasts twelve hours, and releases in twelve hours (Baden n.d.). It is the third key sign of death that may provide yet another ballpark figure for our medical detectives as to time of death. It also offers a clue to what position the person was in when he died. For example, a standing person who is shot to death will fall to the ground, and the development of rigor mortis and livor mortis will reflect that body position. Sometimes rigor mortis will show a person's actions shortly before death. For example, a body may be found in a defensive position with the arms bent upward as if guarding the head. The ME should be able to tell if the decedent was moved after the onset of rigor mortis—as well as livor mortis.

Rigor becomes first noticeable in the face, particularly the jaw, and spreads throughout the body, taking effect in the largest muscles last. In full rigor, the body becomes board-stiff, its joints locked. Rigor's effect is due to a biochemical chain reaction in muscle tissue associated with the cessation of breathing: as oxygen is no longer available to remove calcium from the body's cells, calcium concentration in cells rises. This forces muscles to remain in a contracted state until muscle proteins start to decompose. The body then appears to relax—although in actuality, it is decomposing. After about thirty-six hours, most bodies in rigor will have loosened, the rigor leaving the body in much the same order it took hold.

Many things affect the development of rigor. It progresses relatively slowly in a hot climate and in the obese, as body fat can infiltrate muscle tissue. When a person dies in snow, the rigor that sets in may last until the snow thaws. A study in Torino, Italy, showed that corpses kept at a constant low temperature of 4 degrees Centigrade had a long persistence of rigor mortis that didn't disappear completely until the twenty-eighth day after death—one body stayed in full rigor for sixteen days. The study's cadavers went from complete to partial rigor between the eleventh and seventeenth day after death. All of the bodies studied were in complete rigor by day three (Varetto and Curto 2005).

Fatigue, adrenaline, and high lactic levels in muscle accelerate the onset of rigor. In extreme cases of exertion, this may lead to a phenomenon called "cadaveric spasm." This is what happens: as the person dies, her muscles instantly stiffen in what can be thought of as a form of instant rigor mortis. One example: a drowning person's hands may become rapidly depleted of oxygen and loaded with a buildup of cellular waste as she frantically thrashes to save herself. If she grasped anything along the way, such as reeds at the edge of a river, these may be tightly held in her hand after death.

Due to this depletion of oxygen and accumulation of waste, in general rigor mortis is much more evident sooner in a death following stressful exertion than if the person had died in a relaxed state such as sleep (Baden 2006; Becker 2005; Green, M.A. 2000; Temple 2005; What Is Rigor 2003).

The next process actually begins before rigor mortis, livor mortis, or algor mortis: putrefaction. It may not be immediately obvious, but decay begins quickly after death—within the first four minutes if the body isn't chilled or frozen. Putrefaction's processes are complex, necessary, and mostly due to the hard work of bacteria and enzymes. These physical and chemical changes continue until the body is completely decomposed—with the exception of the bones and hair.

Human decomposition is a process of self-digestion, or *autolysis*. Cells are deprived of oxygen, so carbon dioxide in the blood increases, pH decreases, and wastes accumulate. This is toxic for cells. Meanwhile, unchecked cellular enzymes start dissolving cells from within. Cells respond by disintegrating and let loose their nutrient-rich fluids. As they rupture, rigor mortis begins to relax. Once there's enough nutrient-rich fluid available in the body, putrefaction begins in earnest. This self-digestion accelerates in tissues with high enzyme content, such as in the liver, or with high water content, such as the brain. This process is not usually obvious for a few days (Vass 2001). Through microorganisms such as bacteria, fungi, and protozoa, putrefaction transforms body tissues into gases, liquids, and simple molecules. Bacteria and other microorganisms are already present in the body, but more join in from the immediate environment as well as from visiting flies and other insects.

The earliest sign that putrefaction has begun is a greenish discoloration in the right lower area of the abdomen. This discoloration, due to the breakdown of blood, becomes rapidly apparent throughout the entire abdomen and then the chest. Within four to seven days, surface veins in the limbs become prominent and discolored—an effect known as "marbling." The trunk—especially the bowels—as well as the external genitalia in males and other tissues, including the face and lips, begin to swell with a variety of gases. These include methane, ammonia, sulfur dioxide, hydrogen sulfide, carbon dioxide, and hydrogen. Gas formation is associated with anaerobic fermentation, especially in the gut.

Gas formation in the head presses blood-stained fluid out of the nose and mouth; gas, fluid accumulation, and feces may be forced from the rectum— or can be intense enough to tear abdominal muscles and skin. The skin, meanwhile, acquires a bubbly texture, and blisters filled with pinkish fluid appear. Skin appears loose on the flesh in an effect called "skin slippage"; if touched, large sheets of skin slide off. Body fluids soak into the surroundings. A great deal of gas pressure can build within the body, creating a distended, puffed-up look. This is something police officers often need to contend with as they respond to calls to check on someone's welfare and find a bloated corpse, maybe weeks old.

Once the gas has been purged, active decay starts. The breakdown of amino acids in muscle proteins produces the chemical compound *putrescine* (the odor of this compound makes some vomit), *cadaverine,* and various fatty acids, among other compounds. At this point, aerobic and anaerobic bacteria thrive in large populations, insects are busy feeding and nesting, and scavengers may also be enjoying a free meal.

Not all body parts decompose at the same time. The brain and spleen rapidly liquefy, but the heart and lungs may be visually recognizable for weeks or months. The prostate gland and uterus last even longer—they can be identifiable in remains nearly reduced to bare bones (Anatomic 2004; Green, M.A. 2000; Temple 2005; Vass 2001).

After all the flesh and tissue have broken down, the next step is *desiccation*, a term derived from the Latin word *desiccare,* meaning to dry up completely. In a postmortem context, this refers to the drying that occurs most prominently on mucous membranes (the mucus-producing membrane lining of body cavities that encounter air, such as those of the mouth, lungs, and eyes). A sign of this dessication is *tache noire,* or blackened conjunctiva, the membrane that covers the white part of the eye and lines the inside of the eyeball (Anatomic 2004).

Next, skin and other tissue that survives the active decay process (because it has no nutritional value to organisms) may become dehydrated and mummified. Mummified skin will look like a leathery or paperlike material clinging to the deceased's bones. This happens in dry heat conditions or areas with very low humidity, such as the arctic or desert. Bones go through their own subtler decay process called *diagenesis,* in which they slowly leach organic components, such as collagen, and inorganic compounds, such as calcium, potassium, and magnesium.

Wet environments, meanwhile, can have a completely different effect on corpses. A body in the ocean may be partially eaten by lobsters, starfish, or other marine life or be damaged by boat propellers. Warm, moist conditions can lead to the formation of a yellowish white, greasy waxlike material called *adipocere,* also known as "grave wax" or "mortuary wax." Bodies with adipocere can also be referred to as undergoing "saponification"—the creation of soap from fat in a high pH environment. Adipocere forms when body fat decays in damp or wet anaerobic conditions. It's made up of fatty acids and calcium soaps and results from a process that partially preserves the body: a slow hydrolysis of body fats. Adipocere begins to form several weeks to months after death and can remain for centuries on a body. It inhibits the growth of bacteria. Initially yellowish brown in color and firm, this hydrolyzed fat subsequently whitens and develops an offensive odor. As an aside, adipocere will burn and produce a smoky yellow flame (Green, M.A. 2000; Timmermans 2006; Vass 2001).

A human body's rate of decomposition depends on various environmental conditions, but forensic scientists can use a calculation based on soft tissue decay for a body lying on the ground. For the most part, a body that rots in an environment with an average temperature of 10 degrees Centigrade will be skeletonized (reduced to bones) in about 128 days. Buried bodies and those immersed in water will have different rates depending on conditions. Injuries and skin damage, as well as exposure to scavengers, will increase the rate of decay, as these factors increase bacterial and insect activity. Bones typically bleach within a year and may become a habitat for algae or moss; after ten years they may crack (Vass 2001).

A considerable amount of what is known today about decompositional change in human remains was discovered at the University of Tennessee's Anthropological Research Facility (ARF), otherwise known as "the body farm." This Knoxville facility was founded by esteemed forensic anthropologist Dr. William Bass in the late 1970s, following several cases in which advanced decomposition prevented scientists from estimating time of death. At the time, knowledge of human decomposition was largely anecdotal.

Situated on three acres of land—where bodies lie decaying on the rolling hills of Tennessee—the ARF is the only facility in the world that receives human cadavers to study changes after death. Some of these corpses are donated, while others are unclaimed bodies released by medical examiners. Research efforts cover decomposition rates in a broad mix of settings, such as while hanging, in a car, or in water; testing of body recovery technology; the creation of a photo record of human decay; and the pursuit of biochemical knowledge so scientists may determine a body's "time since death" based on levels of particular gases. Forensic entomologists, cadaver dogs, FBI agents, and others involved in death investigation have also trained and studied at the ARF (Christensen 2006).

Part of what spurred the ARF's creation was a dramatic case of mistaken "time since death" of an initially headless body found in a disturbed Civil War grave in 1977 in Franklin, Tennessee. Dr. Bass, then the head of the University of Tennessee's anthropology department, examined the body and saw a mostly intact, clothed corpse with soft pink tissue. He estimated the person had been dead for about six months to a year, and had been murdered. Police wondered if someone had tried to hide a homicide by burying a body in an old grave. Before long, the head was found. After examining the lack of dental work, as well as other clues such as the clothes' lack of labels and all-natural fiber content, Bass began to have serious doubts about his time-of-death estimate.

Although all other particulars of age, race, sex, and ancestry were correct, the time since death was off—by more than a hundred years. It soon became evident the cadaver was Confederate Colonel William Shy. The colonel had been embalmed, and his solid, hermetically sealed cast-iron coffin had preserved the body against the ravages of decomposition, insects, scavengers, and bacteria. Bass, while embarrassed about his very public error, was intrigued by what clearly wasn't known about human decomposition. The seed for the body farm was sown (Bass and Jefferson 2003; Christensen 2006; Vass 2001).

It can be a grisly subject, but learning about how bodies decay not only helps medical examiners determine time since death but may give clues to the dead person's characteristics—and possibly the person's identity. For example, the amount of fatty acids and other products of decomposition may help to determine the deceased's body weight at death. Trace chemicals or toxins found in the decaying body may help determine cause of death (Vass 2001). Ultimately, it's another key tool in the ME's kit.

3

DEATH AND TRAUMA: SOME
COMMON SIGNS

SIGNS OF TRAUMA can be hard to miss on a body. The physical damage can be due to violence or accident, but from cuts and scrapes to stab wounds and gunshots, these injuries can be dramatic and, in some cases, deadly.

This chapter will cover the types of trauma most commonly encountered in a day's work at the medical examiner's office: abrasions, lacerations, and bruising, as well as variety of unkind cuts, including incised, stab, slash, puncture, and chop wounds. Defense wounds, bite marks, and injuries received from firearms, extreme sexual practices, and other traumas will also be discussed.

There's a great difference between wounds that happen before death and those that happen after. A wound inflicted before death is an *antemortem* wound. When examining a decedent who was alive when the injury was received, the medical examiner will find that white blood cells have moved to the site of the wound to help heal it. Live people can also bleed considerably from stab wounds or other types of cutting injuries. If an artery is hit by a bullet or the edge of a blade, there may be a jet of arterial spray— blood that squirts or spurts from an artery.

Patterns from blood spray made on nearby surfaces depend on the size and severity of the injury, whether the wound was covered with clothes, and the person's position when he was injured. Specialists in this area, called bloodstain pattern analysts, also study drips, transfer patterns, and exhalation patterns—all in all, any geometry made by moving blood. At a death scene indoors, spray patterns can sometimes be seen on several walls and also on the ceiling. A person may have coughed up blood; someone untrained in bloodstain pattern analysis might think this spray was produced by a gunshot wound.

Bleeding also occurs under the skin in live people. If, for example, a rope or other material tied around the wrist ruptures a small blood vessel in a living victim without breaking the skin, there will be internal hemorrhaging and blood will spill into surrounding tissue (Temple 2005; Turvey 2002).

Traumas inflicted after death—or *postmortem* wounds—usually create very little or no bleeding from broken arteries and veins. As the heart is not pumping, and therefore not moving the blood, there's no pressure to generate spray. Bruises are another matter. In some injuries, it can take twenty-four to forty-eight hours for the blood leaking into tissues to be visible on the surface; thus, a bruise may appear after death, and possibly even after the autopsy. Other bruises may appear more pronounced. Generally, dead tissue does not swell or bruise as a result of injury, although there are exceptions. If a dead body is hit with enough force soon after death, what resembles bruising may appear—but the mark will likely be disproportionately small compared to the impact. Some researchers have called this "pseudo bruising." Also, lesions that look like pre-death bruises can appear in the neck muscles of a body while the neck organs undergo autopsy.

The very act of performing an autopsy will create some of these pseudo bruises and make actual antemortem bruises migrate—a fact a forensic pathologist needs to be aware of if performing a second autopsy. These post-death bruises usually show less hemorrhage into tissue than bruises inflicted in live tissue, but in some cases may be difficult to distinguish from antemortem bruises (Langlois and Gresham 1991; Temple 2005; Turvey 2002; Vanezis 2001).

The discoloration of bruises is also referred to as *ecchymosis*. The word *contusion* is also used for bruising, particularly in deeper injuries. In a live body, the color of the bruise changes as hemoglobin in the injury degrades, fading from blue to brown, green, and yellow until it disappears. Bruising is much easier to see in fairer-skinned people, so medical examiners have to take care not to overlook bruising in people with deeper skin tones. Contusions are usually caused by a blow to the body, and may be located on the surface of the skin or internally, such as on the brain or heart. In some cases, bruising may be part of a disease process, or, if blood has moved away from the impact area, the bruise may be seen at a site away from the injury (Vanezis 2001).

It may be possible to match a bruise with the object that caused it, such as the heel of a shoe, and thus help build a picture of what happened to the decedent. Some objects produce typical bruises: fingertips may create round or disc-like small bruises, while long, cylindrical objects such as a baseball bat create tramline bruising. An ME may also surmise that handcuffs may have produced contusions circling wrists or ankles (Vanezis 2001).

Tissue density determines how easily and fast an area will bruise—it's relatively difficult to bruise the sole of the feet, but fairly easy to bruise the neck. Areas with loose tissue, such as the eyelids, bruise easily after minor trauma. A deep thigh bruise may not appear for a day or two and may look fresh when it finally emerges, while a bruise on the eyebrow will appear very quickly. The age and physical condition of a person can also affect how they bruise. Persons with blood disorders are prone to bruising, and elderly persons and children with loosely supported vasculature (network of blood vessels) bruise more easily than young adults. Bruises last longer in older people, too (Anatomic 2004; Fatteh 1973; Knight 1997; Turvey 2002).

When examining bruises, the forensic pathologist takes into account all factors affecting how a person may bruise: age, physical condition, and where the injury is located. He must confirm that the mark is indeed a bruise before he considers how it may have been made and when—any answers may be very helpful to a death investigation. Dating a bruise by its color can be misleading, however, because of all the variables that affect bruising, as well as the unavoidable level of subjectivity involved in a naked-eye examination.

Some bruises can indicate dangerous habits. As regular witnesses to the end result of illegal drug use, medical examiners are well aware that illicit drugs are widely used throughout society. One sign suggesting illegal drug use is numerous bruise-like needle marks on the arms or legs or between toes (Genge 2002).

Abrasions are another common type of trauma. In this injury, friction wears off layers of outer skin (or epidermis). Depending on the severity of the scrape or abrasion in a live person, the wound may bleed and seep serum (the protein-rich fluid in blood that remains when platelets coagulate) as a protective scab or crust forms. A tangential impact that skids across the skin produces most abrasions. A body that is dragged or pushed across a rough surface like concrete will also have abrasions. Other marks can be mistaken for abrasions on a body, such as the chew marks of cockroaches (Temple 2005).

Abrasions are important to the medical examiner because they retain the pattern of what produced them. It may be possible to link a specific patterned wound to any number of things, including the bumper of a car. Such was the case for a murder committed via automobile in Texas. In July 2002, married couple Clara and David Harris, both forty-four-year-old dentists, had an argument at the Nassau Bay Hilton because of David Harris's affair with his dental receptionist. In the parking lot afterward, Clara Harris struck her unfaithful husband with her Mercedes, knocking him twenty-five feet. She crossed two medians and ran over him at least two more times, then put the car into reverse and backed over him. David Harris died at Christus St. John Hospital fourteen minutes after arrival.

David Harris's body was taken to the Harris County Medical Examiner's Office in Houston. He had cuts on his scalp and abrasions on his head and neck. His lungs, punctured by ribs, had collapsed. His jaw, pelvis, and back were broken, every rib fractured. His vena cava, the vein through which blood flows back to the heart, was torn, as was his bladder. The ME who performed the autopsy determined that a crushed chest was the cause of death.

After deliberating five hours on Valentine's Day 2003, a jury found Clara Harris guilty of murder. Judge Carol Davies sentenced her to twenty years in prison and levied a $10,000 fine. Harris was incarcerated at the Mountain View Unit, Texas Department of Corrections, in Gatesville on September 16, 2003 (Long 2004).

Abrasions from kicking are commonly seen in homicides and assaults. Usually the perpetrator is wearing shoes and the victim is attacked while lying on the ground. The kicks typically land on the victim's face, neck, side of chest, and side of the abdomen. Yet the kicker may leave behind potentially incriminating evidence. A perpetrator who stomps on his victim's back can produce a compression abrasion of footwear treads. A medical examiner may work with a tread expert witness to match up the marks with a high degree of credibility, especially if the ME and tread expert testify in court. An abrasion not visible on wet skin may be noticeable after the body has been in the morgue cooler for a day (Anatomic 2004; Knight 1997; Turvey 2002).

A tear in the skin—or laceration—is produced by friction or impact with a blunt object over an area with a bony structure underneath—for example, the scalp, face, and knees. A laceration bleeds profusely and its edges may be ragged, bruised, and abraded. As an aside, a bullet that strikes the skin tangentially or strikes it at a single point without penetrating the skin can make the skin appear as if it were lacerated (Anatomic 2004; Knight 1997; Turvey 2002).

Actor William Holden's death illustrates how a laceration can be a killer. Holden, who appeared in almost seventy movies between 1939 and 1981, including *Sunset Boulevard* and *The Towering Inferno*, was a private person who was living alone when he died in 1981. He lived at Shorecliff Towers, 535 Ocean Avenue, Apartment 43, in Santa Monica, California.

On November 16, Bill Martin, the apartment building manager, used a passkey to enter Holden's apartment because he had not seen Holden for a number of days and was concerned about the actor's welfare. In the suite, all the lights were off and the television was on. Holden, wearing a pajama top, shirt, and underwear, was lying on the floor beside his bed. He had a deep laceration in his forehead. The carpet, his clothes, and the bed sheets were soaked in blood from the injury. Eight bloodied Kleenex tissues were on the bed. The heavy teakwood table next to the bed had been moved, and one corner of the table had produced a gash in the wall. There were drops of blood on the nearby telephone. In the kitchen, an empty bottle of vodka and four beer bottles sat in the trash can, and a partially full bottle of vodka rested in the sink. Martin and others who knew Holden were aware he had a drinking problem.

Dr. Thomas T. Noguchi, Los Angeles chief medical examiner, performed the autopsy. He observed maggots in the eyes and mouth, a dehydrated finger, dry blood on both hands, skin slippage on one arm and on one leg, and decomposed genital organs. Rigor mortis, body temperature, decomposition, cloudy eyes, and a greenish abdomen indicated to Noguchi that Holden had been dead at least four days before Martin found the body.

Toxicological data indicated Holden's blood alcohol was 0.22 percent—more than double the legal definition of driving under the influence of alcohol in California. Noguchi determined Holden bled to death because of the depth of the actor's two-and-a-half-inch head laceration, compounded by the effects of alcohol. The intoxicant dilates capillaries, contributes to bleeding, and inhibits blood clotting in open wounds.

Noguchi concluded that Holden was intoxicated before he died, and that he tripped on the throw rug in the bedroom, lunged forward, and struck his head on the corner of the table—the force of impact driving the corner of the table into the wall. Holden, still conscious, opened the drawer of the table, removed Kleenex, and attempted to stem the flow of blood from the forehead laceration. He likely lost consciousness after half an hour. Noguchi deemed the manner of death accidental, as there was no sign of forced entry, no indication of robbery, and no evidence of any weapons (Anatomic 2004; Noguchi 1983; Thomas 1983; Turvey 2002; William Holden 2004).

A wide variety of weapons can create wounds that break the skin, from axes and butcher knives to sewing shears and knitting needles. All inflict their own type of damage, leaving clues for the observant medical examiner. Stab wounds are made when a pointed instrument such as a knife, scissors, or chisel pierces the skin and often the underlying tissue. The depth of the piercing usually creates more injury to the underlying tissue than to the surface of the skin, where the pointed instrument first makes contact. The most common bodily targets of stabbings are the chest or abdomen (Knight 1997; Turvey 2002). An incised wound is a cut made by a sharp, bladelike object drawn across the surface of the skin or into the flesh. This wound tends to be longer than it is deep. Both serrated and non-serrated blades produce the same type of smooth edges (Anatomic 2004; Turvey 2002).

One case involving various cutting wounds had audiences in the early 1990s glued to their TV screens across America. Nicole Brown Simpson, murdered in Los Angeles in June 1994, suffered a vicious incised wound on her neck—although multiple sharp force injuries or stabbing caused her death. Her husband, the football star and actor O.J. Simpson, was charged with her murder. Although he was acquitted after a criminal trial, he was found guilty in a civil trial (Golden 1994). O.J. Simpson was also charged with the murder of Ron Goldman, Nicole Brown Simpson's friend, whose body was found not far from hers. Goldman had multiple stab wounds in his chest, abdomen, and left thigh—his death was also caused by multiple sharp force injuries (Golden 1994). As in Nicole Brown Simpson's case, O.J. Simpson was acquitted after a criminal trial and found guilty after a civil trial.

The civil trial pitted two respected forensic pathologists' opinions against each other: Dr. Michael Baden, former chief medical examiner of New York City, testified for the defense, and Dr. Werner Spitz served as expert for the plaintiffs (the families of Brown Simpson and Goldman). Spitz asserted that the two victims' fingernails made the cuts on O.J. Simpson's hand during the attack; Baden said he believed Simpson's explanation that he cut himself on broken glass after the murders, according to a December 17, 1996, article in the *New York Times*, "Expert for Simpson Disputes Testimony on Cuts."

Among other key points of disagreement covered in the article, Baden said the killer should have had blood splatter on his clothes, while Spitz said the killer could have left the scene clean of blood due to the killer's position during the attacks. The defense also provided the testimony of a blood splatter expert, who suggested that blood was planted on socks found on Simpson's bed after the murders. This case illustrates how forensic experts can vastly differ over the same evidence.

Slash wounds, another type of cut wound, are longer than they are deep. This type of wound is often inflicted during a knife fight while the participants move about, tangentially slicing each other. In general, a slash wound is much less dangerous to a victim than a stab wound, unless a victim is slashed in the face or neck (Knight 1997). If one of the fight's participants had an axe, meat cleaver, or another sharp-edged, heavy instrument, however, his opponent could suffer a nasty chop wound. This is a deep tissue injury and often includes bone fractures (Turvey 2002).

Like a stab wound, a puncture wound is a penetrating injury made by an object with a point, such as an ice pick, and tends to have more depth than width. A puncture wound running right through an organ is also referred to as a perforating wound. Puncture wounds can create considerable internal bleeding, although an inexperienced person looking at the entry point on the skin's surface may conclude the wound is not serious or life threatening. Massive hemorrhage is usually the cause of death with this type of wound (Anatomic 2004; Lerner and Lerner 2006).

The shape of stab or cutting wounds offers some information, too. A wound shaped like the letters "L," "Y," or "V" occurs when a knife blade plunged into the body is twisted before the knife is pulled out, or when the victim turns while the knife is in the body. A hilt mark or imprint abrasion shows the perpetrator shoved the knife into the victim up to the end of the blade. A wound cut to resemble a pentagram, a five-pointed star, suggests the perpetrator has a connection to a satanic cult.

A victim's injuries are described as defense wounds when the victim receives them while trying to defend himself. These wounds are defined further as being "active" or "passive," as their positioning may offer information about the attack. For example, a stabbing victim may suffer an active defense wound on the palm of his hand if he grasps the knife his attacker is thrusting at him. Or, he may endure passive defense wounds on his arms or hands if he raises them to protect himself against his attacker. A victim may also have active defense wounds on his legs if he was in a lying position and kicked the perpetrator, or passive defense wounds if he curled up in the fetal position in an attempt to protect his body with his legs. A victim can also receive defense wounds when attempting to deflect kicks, fists, or blunt instruments—or any kind of attack. These injuries will mostly be seen on the decedent's hands, wrists, or forearms, but can also be on the thighs if the victim is attempting to shield his groin from kicks. Sometimes a blunt instrument, such as a hammer, glass bottle, gun, or baseball bat, used to injure someone will leave trace material behind in a laceration. This can help police identify the weapon (Pollak and Saukko 2000).

One type of weapon is almost always present: teeth. A pair of curved, opposing bruises characterize the human bite mark, but may also include laceration, a crushing of tissues, and some tearing away of skin and flesh. Human bite marks are most often seen in sexual assaults—heterosexual and homosexual—as well as in homicides, domestic violence, and child abuse. In sexual assaults, these marks are usually made on the side of the victim's neck, shoulders, and breasts, especially in the nipple area. Bites are also seen on the nose, ears, and lips. On children, bite marks are commonly inflicted on the arms and buttocks.

Bite marks, tool marks, and fingerprints all have their own qualities. If a bite mark is clear, this type of evidence can be significant, as sets of teeth often have qualities that make them unique: the alignment, size, shape, and damage, as well as any dental work. Even identical twins have distinctive individual teeth. A forensic odontologist, a specialist in evaluating dental evidence, uses her skills to identify human remains from dental records, make age estimations, and identify child abuse. Although there is still some debate about using bite marks as evidence due to concerns about accuracy and subjectivity, this type of evidence helped convict one of the country's most notorious killers.

On Super Bowl Sunday 1978, at the Chi Omega sorority house at Florida State University, in Tallahassee, serial killer Ted Bundy murdered two sleeping coeds and badly injured two others. He bit victim Lisa Levy once on the breast and twice on the buttocks. Bite mark evidence linked him to her murder, and he was sentenced to death in Florida's electric chair. Bundy was executed in 1989 (Miletich 2003).

If an ME sees what he thinks are bite marks, he will ask a forensic odontologist to confirm that the mark is indeed from a bite and, if so, if it's possible to determine the tooth pattern of the perpetrator. The forensic odontologist takes photographs of the visible bite marks and uses ultraviolet or infrared light to expose faint or hidden bite marks. Like bruises, bite mark patterns in living and deceased individuals change over time. For this reason, the forensic odontologist may have to examine bite mark evidence more than once to note and photograph changes in the pattern.

Tissue around bite marks should not be disturbed when handling the body because this could distort them. If the body must be moved before bite mark or saliva evidence is obtained, a small piece of cardboard or sturdy paper can be secured over the bite mark to protect any saliva surrounding the mark. One way to collect this evidence is to moisten a sterile cotton swab with sterile saline or distilled water and to gently swab the skin in a circular motion, starting from the center of the bite mark. The swab is labeled and set aside to air dry. A second dry swab is used to repeat the procedure. For control purposes, the procedure is repeated at a site where there is no bite mark. The three swabs become part of the chain of custody.

Investigators will compare DNA evidence from the bite marks to samples from any suspects. They may collect saliva for DNA testing from a suspect by having the suspect deposit saliva on a clean piece of filter paper until the wet mark is two inches in diameter. The mark is then circled with a pencil and air-dried before it is submitted to a lab. Matching the suspect's saliva with the victim's bite mark solidly links the two.

Incidentally, the first time bite mark evidence was used to convict a criminal was in 1906 in England. Investigators compared a bite mark on cheese at the scene of a burglary to the bite mark of a suspect. The bite marks matched and the burglar was convicted (Gray-Ray, Hensley, and Brennan 1997; Knight 1997; Williams 2003).

Occasionally, a dead person will be found to have bitten himself. The usual locations of these bites are the sides of the tongue. A fresh bite mark indicates that a seizure may have preceded the person's death. A bite mark may be the only anatomical evidence to suggest that an epileptic died during an epileptic attack (Spitz 1980).

Not all bite marks found on bodies are made by humans, of course. Dogs, cats, ferrets, gerbils, raccoons, rats, bats, bears—the list of potential biters continues. The injuries, however, are usually quite different in size and distribution from human bites. Dog bites typically have puncture wounds where the four canine teeth have perforated the skin. A dog's incisors are small and rarely leave a mark in minor nips. More serious dog bites can involve punctures inflicted when the dog grasps its victim in its mouth; cuts from the gripping action of the dog's incisors; and tissue loss caused by the dog's premolars and molars. The victim may also suffer lesions if the attacking dog drags him and shakes its head while biting. An investigator can determine if more than one dog was involved in the attack by measuring inter-canine widths—the width between the canine teeth.

Ferrets are becoming popular as pets in the U.S., yet these animals can be hazardous, particularly to small children. Ferrets may bite and scratch without provocation; they may regard infants as prey and can inflict serious wounds very rapidly. A 2007 case report in France notes how a six-week-old infant lost 60 percent of the external part of an ear to an attack by his parents' pet ferret. Ferrets also may carry potentially deadly contagious diseases such as rabies, tuberculosis, and flu (Ferrant, Papin, Du Pont, Jr., Clin, and Babin 2008). Ferret bites can look like rat bites, but rats are less likely to attack a live, screaming child or person.

Rats and other rodents will bite corpses, however. These animals inflict damage that looks round and crater-like, with chewed irregular edges. There also may be puncture wounds, scrapes, and lacerations from their sharp incisors. Tissue or cartilage may be missing. Rodents will usually bite exposed and unprotected parts of the body—for example, the back of the hands and moist parts of the face: eyelids, nose, and mouth (Ferrant, Papin, Du Pont, Jr., Clin, and Babin 2008).

In snakes, the appearance of the bite depends on the viciousness of the snake; in venomous snake bites one can see isolated fang punctures, while non-venomous snakes leave multiple scratch-like teeth marks on skin (Whittaker 1994).

Another type of bite-like mark is known as a "love bite," or petechial hemorrhage. These flat, tiny, round purplish red spots are often made during consensual sexual activity or in assaults. Caused by suction and seen with or without a surrounding bite mark, petechial hemorrhages are typically found on the neck or chest. Children and adolescents sometimes inflict similar marks on arms. These hemorrhages range from two-tenths of a millimeter to two millimeters in size and are produced by blood vessels rupturing. When something prevents congested blood from returning to the heart, the tiny, blood-engorged venules leak blood into surrounding areas (Wecht, Saitz, and Curriden 2003).

Some sexual practices can result in unusual and potentially dangerous injuries that a medical examiner may need to identify. In fisting, also known as handballing, one partner inserts his hand into his partner's anus, usually with the help of a lot of lubrication. Prior to insertion, participants may use marijuana or a sedative-hypnotic drug, such as methaqualone, to help them relax. They may also take a vasodilator such as amyl nitrite as a muscle relaxant. Injuries associated with fisting include rectosigmoid perforations, or holes in the sigmoid colon and the upper part of the rectum, and anal sphincter lacerations, possibly producing anal incontinence. Some men die of complications from anal fisting trauma, some women from vaginal fisting trauma. Homicide is the manner of death in some cases (Cohen, Giles, and Nelson 2004; Fain and McCormick 1989; Handballing 2006; Reay and Eisele 1983).

Another potentially deadly sexual activity is autoerotic asphyxia, done with rope, cords, or some other ligature. In this practice, the typically solo participant partially strangles himself to enhance his sexual experience. He may suspend himself indoors from a beam or outdoors from a tree branch and, while masturbating, attempt to regulate the pressure around his neck to decrease the amount of oxygen reaching his brain. The decrease in oxygen available to the brain (cerebral hypoxia) is said to enhance sexual stimulation and orgasm; usually the asphyxiation is meant to be brief and non-fatal. However, the individual may slip, the rope around his neck may become too tight, and he may asphyxiate. The result: accidental death.

The manner of death can also be suicide, homicide, or natural. For example, a person not able to free herself from the rope may be a victim of a sexually related homicide if evidence suggests the deceased was not alone. A death due to autoerotic asphyxia may be ruled as a suicide rather than an accident, depending on circumstances and evidence. Regardless, this type of death is difficult for families and friends, and embarrassed relatives may not always cooperate with investigators.

White males under the age of thirty have historically represented the majority of those who have died from this activity. Females are usually found naked with one ligature and no unusual equipment. Some adult males participate with a partner and engage in homosexual sadomasochistic behavior. Practitioners commonly use pornographic materials; some cross-dress. Instead of hanging from a rope, others fit a plastic bag over their heads, inhale noxious chemicals, such as butae and nitrous oxide, or partially or totally submerge themselves in water (Beattie 2005; Byard and Bramwell 1991; Byard, Hucker, and Hazelwood 1990; Newton 1998; Shields, Hunsaker, D.M., and Hunsaker, J.C., III 2005; Wesselius and Bally 1983).

In addition to regularly examining injuries from sharp and blunt instruments, forensic pathologists often see firearm wounds. The appearance of these wounds can offer valuable information about the shooting. Often the medical examiner will consult a ballistics expert in a firearms case.

It used to be commonly accepted that all entrance wounds are small, puncture-type holes, while exit wounds are bigger with jagged edges. Research has shown this is not always the case. Generally, an exit wound is larger and more irregular than an entrance wound, but on occasion it may be identical to or smaller than the entrance wound (Apfelbaum, Shockley, Wahe, and Moore 1998).

One clear sign of an entrance wound is an abrasion ring—a ring of damaged tissue around the wound where the bullet scraped the skin as it entered the body. Other signs of an entrance wound depend on how far the victim was from the gun when he was shot. For example, a hard contact wound is made when the muzzle of a gun is pressed firmly against the skin and fired. The skin circling the wound will be embedded with soot, a by-product of burned gunpowder and vaporized metals. Hot gases released from the gun will also sear the edge of the entrance wound. The gases burn, stretch, and rip the skin, making triangular tears and possibly giving the wound an irregular shape (Apfelbaum, Shockley, Wahe, and Moore 1998).

A gun muzzle held lightly against the skin creates a loose contact wound; its soot ring can easily be wiped away. A victim could also have an angled contact wound, made when the gun is held at an angle to the skin. This leaves a pear-shaped mark with seared skin and soot on the opposite side of the gun barrel. Other possibilities include near-contact wounds, made from about an inch away characterized by a larger circle of scorched skin and soot; angled near-contact wounds, evident by soot and irregular seared skin on the same side as the barrel; intermediate-range wounds, marked by gunpowder injuries called "tattooing"; and distant wounds, not marked by anything but the injury itself.

Tattooing is produced when gunpowder grains disperse rapidly from enough distance to spray out and become embedded in the skin. Tattooing looks like red or brown lesions scattered around the entrance wound and is not considered a powder burn. Only muzzle-loading weapons that use black powder can cause a powder burn. These emit white smoke and flame and can burn skin or set the victim's clothes on fire. Sometimes insect bites produce changes in the skin and create pseudo-tattooing. Likewise, material that looks like soot and is deposited on the skin is pseudo-soot.

Exit wounds do not show soot or tattooing. The appearance of the exit wound depends on the deformation and instability of a bullet as it passes through the body. In a skull, a typical entrance wound has a clean, punched-out external appearance and a round or ovoid shape. A skull exit wound is usually more irregular and is almost always larger than the entrance wound. It will also have an inward, punched-out appearance (Apfelbaum, Shockley, Wahe, and Moore 1998; Quatrehomme and Iscan 1998; Smock 2000; Zaki and Hanzlick 1987).

New technology can be hazardous. One controversial cause of death that was first noted in the 1990s is death from Taser. These devices are hand-held battery-powered weapons, also known as conductive energy devices or stun guns, and are used to subdue aggressive people who disobey police commands. Tasers have been manufactured since 1993 in Scottsdale, Arizona, by Taser International, the world's largest manufacturer of stun guns. More than 7,000 law enforcement agencies throughout the U.S. use these weapons. An officer who uses this device, rather than a baton or police dog, does not have to be close to his target and so will struggle less with him. Carrying a Taser can therefore prevent injury to the officer as well as the person to be subdued, as well as reduce the need for a gun.

The typical non-compliant person is a young unarmed male who acts in a bizarre way due to the effects of alcohol or some other intoxicant. This person may show symptoms of a psychological disorder, including hallucinations, and may jump on top of a police car or smash through a plate glass window. When an officer activates his Taser, compressed nitrogen delivers a five-second, 50,000-volt jolt of electricity. This happens after an electrical signal is transmitted through two insulated wires, each with a probe at its end; in seconds the probe travels up to twenty-five feet and makes contact with the target. The person loses neuromuscular control as well as the ability to perform coordinated action for the duration of the impulse.

The controversy regarding Taser is whether this weapon causes the death of very agitated people that police attempt to subdue, or if Taser plays only a part in these deaths, or whether the device is not at all responsible. In

2005, in Chicago, Illinois, the Cook County Medical Examiner's Office reported that two Taser jolts delivered by a Chicago police officer caused death by electrocution of fifty-four-year-old Ronald Hasse earlier that year. Hasse, a former securities trader, was to have been on trial in June regarding a buried body on an Indiana farm. During a confrontation with Hasse, police used a Taser device after Hasse attempted to kick and bite officers and threatened to infect paramedics with HIV. Hasse's death was the first time a medical examiner reported that Taser was the *primary* cause of death. Until then, some coroners and medical examiners reported that Taser contributed to some deaths. In Hasse's case, methamphetamines contributed to his demise.

Taser International used to maintain that excited delirium is the cause of death in people who die after a Taser jolt. *Excited delirium* is a term associated with the widespread cocaine use, perhaps at an epidemic level, during the 1980s and with people who mysteriously died while in police custody. Dr. Deborah Mash, a brain researcher, examined the brains of people identified as excited delirium victims and found that almost all of these victims had abused drugs—usually cocaine or amphetamine. In 2005, the Taser manufacturer stated that a medical examiner has never cited Taser as the sole cause of death.

In February 2005, James Ruggieri, a forensic engineer, said in his presentation to the American Academy of Forensic Sciences that Taser shocks could cause delayed ventricular fibrillation, a form of cardiac arrest. It's marked by a series of rapid, uncoordinated contractions throughout the lower chambers of the heart that prevent blood from being pumped. Sudden unconsciousness is usually the only symptom, and the afflicted person will die unless the normal rhythm of the heart is restored.

From 1999 until July 2005, 140 cases of death in the U.S. and Canada were connected to police Taser shock. As of 2005, Taser International was facing at least twenty lawsuits claiming wrongful death or injury (Anglen 2006; Briscoe 2005; Excited 2003; Kornblum 1991).

Another type of trauma medical examiners see is Shaken Baby Syndrome (SBS), a type of child abuse specific to infants. As its name implies, this syndrome is seen in a baby who has been violently shaken or whose head has struck a hard surface. The resulting trauma includes brain hemorrhage, retinal hemorrhage, rib fractures, and bruises, and can lead to serious brain injury or death. Boys appear to be victims slightly more often than girls.

American radiologist John Caffey described injuries associated with this syndrome in 1946. He noted fractures in the long bones (such as the thighs) of infants suffering from subdural hematomas, and bleeding between the outer protective covering of the brain and the middle fibrous membrane that covers the brain and spinal cord. In 1971, British neurosurgeon A.N. Guthkelch first described the association between subdural hematomas and whiplash injuries in infants and the possible mechanism of injury.

In 1974, Caffey coined the expression *Whiplash Shaken Infant Syndrome* (WSIS). Some experts prefer the term *Shaken Impact Syndrome* (SIS) because this term emphasizes the cranial impact that causes severe brain injury in some victims of SBS.

Perpetrators of SBS tend to be inadequately prepared for caring for children and include, among others, parents, live-in boyfriends, stepparents, and grandparents. An incident of SBS typically occurs when a baby begins to cry and a caregiver grabs the baby under the arms and violently shakes the infant, causing the baby's head to rapidly whip back and forth. Acceleration, deceleration, and rotational forces cause veins in the brain to stretch and tear as the brain moves in the cranial cavity. Acceleration-deceleration forces shear the vitreous humor of the eye away from the retina and produce hemorrhaging.

Babies are especially susceptible to acceleration-deceleration injuries because of their large head size relative to their small bodies, as well as their weak neck muscles. The baby's ribs may also fracture when the caregiver grabs and shakes the infant, compressing the ribcage. In twenty seconds, a caregiver may shake a baby from forty to fifty times. The caregiver may then throw the baby into its crib or onto a bed, causing skull fractures when the baby's head hits a solid surface. The caregiver may not be identified as a perpetrator of SBS because there may be no external injuries, no witnesses to the incident, and no admission by the caregiver that he or she shook the infant. In some cases, there is no external evidence of SBS in a baby until the baby dies and an autopsy is performed. Magnetic resonance imaging (MRI) can be used to confirm an SBS injury (Blumenthal 2002; Fulton 2000; Nakagawa and Conway, Jr. 2004).

People of all ages can be hurt in seemingly infinite ways. But while medical examiners are alert for signs of trauma, it's not enough simply to identify injuries. The ME must determine if the trauma he detects on a body did in fact contribute to the death of the deceased.

4

---·-·---

DEATH BY HOSTILE ENVIRONMENT

A KEY ASPECT of medical examiner work is the role of public health officer. Human life may be fragile, but an ME can have a positive impact on people's health and well-being. As medical examiners see many tragic, preventable deaths, much of their work tends to focus on prevention as well as advocacy and education.

Yet there will always be those who do not, or cannot, step out of harm's way. Or perhaps they take a wrong turn on a snowy road in winter and fail to realize it until it is too late. In this chapter, we'll look at the deadly effects the immediate environment can have on a person's health.

Cold can be a killer. Basic human survival requires a body temperature within a fairly tight range. Humans and other warm-blooded animals have internally regulated temperatures that are almost constant for specific time periods, regardless of the temperature of the surrounding air. But human beings—unlike, for example, polar bears—do not have enough hair to keep them warm outdoors. If a person has not dressed adequately, more heat escapes from his body than his body can produce. This creates a dangerous deficit.

Body heat can be lost in several ways: evaporation, if the person has perspired; conduction, if the person sits on cold ground; convection, when cool air circulates around a person; radiation, when heat radiates from a person; and respiration, from the person's breath. If unchecked, heat dissipation results in death.

The body compensates for decreases in temperature by contracting blood vessels close to the surface of the skin. This reduces blood flow to the extremities (where cold air would cool the blood) and keeps the body's core warm. If a person's temperature drops from the normal 98.6 to 96 degrees Fahrenheit, he may shiver visibly and his ability to perform complex tasks will be impaired. If his temperature drops to between 95 and 91 degrees, he will shiver violently. If his body temperature drops below 90 degrees, he's reached a dangerously low body temperature. This is hypothermia. His skin now looks blue and puffy, his body movements become uncontrolled, and his shivering will be replaced by muscular rigidity. At body temperatures dropping to between 85 and 81 degrees, he has pain in exposed parts of his body and difficulty breathing. If this unfortunate person's temperature drops below 78 degrees, his heart will abruptly stop functioning and he will die.

People most likely to experience hypothermia include the very old; the chronically ill, especially those with heart problems; and those under the influence of alcohol or drugs. Falling off a boat into cold water as well as not drinking enough or eating enough in cold weather can also cause hypothermia. In immersion hypothermia—dangerously low body temperature in water—death occurs rapidly, most frequently from drowning as the person's cold limbs soon lose any ability to swim. Some people who have died from hypothermia while indoors have been found under a bed or in closet while partially or completely undressed. This burrowing-like behavior may be an attempt at self-protection, similar to hibernating animals (Rothschild and Schneider 1995).

Autopsies on those who died on land due to cold—dry hypothermia—often reveal gastric mucosal erosions called Wischnewski ulcers. These ulcers, usually shallow with diameters of approximately 0.1 to 0.5 centimeters, are approximately the same distance from each other and form a series of lines (Birchmeyer and Mitchell 1989; Decker 2005; Environmental 2005; Hirvonen 2000; Hypothermia 2005).

A recent case of hypothermia death in the wilderness of southern Oregon made headlines across the country in November and December of 2006. On November 25, James Kim, a thirty-five-year-old senior editor for CNET.com, was driving his Saab station wagon with his wife and two children to San Francisco from Portland, after spending Thanksgiving in Seattle. They intended to stay at a resort in Gold Beach, but took a wrong turn after missing the Highway 42 interchange from Highway 5.

Kim and his wife, Kati Kim, thirty, and daughters Penelope, four, and Sabine, seven months, drove down a narrow road used by loggers, stopped to spend the night, then endured seven days in the car during rain and snowfall. The Kims burned magazines, branches, and a tire for heat. After they drank their last bottle of water, they made more by melting snow. They ate baby food, jelly, and berries; Kati Kim breastfed the girls. Finally, James Kim built a fire for Kati Kim and the children and then set out on foot to get help, leaving a trail of discarded clothing and pieces of a map as clues for searchers. His tennis shoes were inappropriate for a snowy hike. On December 6, a helicopter pilot spotted James Kim's fully clothed body in a creek in the Big Windy Creek ravine. His choice of direction was a tragic and unlucky mistake; a fishing lodge sat only about a mile from where their station wagon was parked. The deputy state medical examiner for southern Oregon, Dr. James Olson, performed the autopsy and confirmed that James Kim died of hypothermia and exposure. Kati Kim and the children were rescued on Monday, December 6 (Kim 2006; Sulek 2006).

Cold can have curious effects on people. One of the strangest is known as "paradoxical undressing." Although the temperature outdoors may be at the freezing point or lower, some people feel compelled to undress—removing a few pieces or all of their clothing. These people feel hot when others feel cold. A number will die of hypothermia. There is no commonly accepted explanation for paradoxical undressing. One theory involves the thermoregulatory center of the brain, the area associated with regulating body temperature. Apparently, this area of the brain is excited by oxides of adrenaline, a hormone released by the body in reaction to stress to prepare the body for "flight" or "fight." The person's metabolism increases and she feels abnormally hot, even to the point that she hallucinates.

Men and women are found dead and inappropriately dressed in open-area, outside locations in the U.S., Canada, Japan, Sweden, Denmark, and other countries where outdoor temperatures can drop to freezing or lower temperatures. Heart disease, alcoholism, and psychotropic drugs (drugs used to treat psychological illnesses) are commonly associated with these people.

Paradoxical undressing can mislead those who are first on the scene of a death from exposure. For example, a person who finds a dead woman who has paradoxically undressed may believe the woman was sexually assaulted and murdered. This conclusion may be based, in part, on the garments near the woman's body—sometimes a trail of clothes leads to the corpse. An experienced police officer or medical examiner would not assume this victim died of sexual assault and murder. An ME who could not be certain at a scene would confirm cause and manner of death at an autopsy.

Dr. Harald Gormsen, University Institute of Forensic Medicine in Copenhagen, Denmark, investigated a case of paradoxical undressing in 1963. On the morning of January 16, a thirty-seven-year-old woman was found dead in a forest. She was lying naked in a prone position, frozen stiff, a wristwatch on her left wrist, her clothing around her body. She had some scratches on her back, but investigators saw no indication of a struggle involving her and any other person at the scene. Only two sets of human footprints were visible: the woman's footprints and the footprints of the person who discovered her body.

Her brother identified the body and told police his sister, who was feeling depressed, had left her parents' home and then disappeared. Her doctor, who said she had a history of depression, prescribed chlorpromazine and meprobamate for her a few days prior to her death. Chlorpromazine is an antipsychotic and tranquilizing agent; meprobamate, a sedative and tranquilizer. The autopsy revealed that animals were probably responsible after her death for the scratches on her back. She had meprobamate in her blood and liver. The autopsy found no indication of strangulation, sperm in her vagina, or pregnancy. The cause of death was freezing; the manner of death was undetermined.

The discovery in 1991 of the Ice Man, a mummified 5,300-year-old body in a glacier in Austria, may be evidence that paradoxical undressing is a phenomenon thousands of years old. The Ice Man's body was found face-down in a shallow depression. He was stripped to the waist, his clothing, believed to be a robe, at his legs. The glacier had passed over the top of the depression and could not have torn away the robe. Instead the Ice Man himself removed the robe, according to Edda Ambach, a forensic scientist at the University of Innsbruck, Austria.

Many people who freeze to death are found prone like the Ice Man: their bodies shut down with the cold, their minds become confused, and they crawl prior to their death (Carey, Griffin, Mason, and Weiss 1993; Gormsen 1972; Mizukami, Shimizu, Shiono, Uezono, and Sasaki 1999; Sivaloganathan 1986; Wedin, Vanggaard, and Hirvonen 1979).

From deadly cold to hazardous heat: the next extreme is death by fire. The majority of fire-related deaths are accidental; the victims are frequently very young or old, as they have the most difficulty escaping. Faulty electrical wiring, faulty electrical appliances, and carelessness with matches and lit cigarettes cause these fires.

An example: A person falls asleep while smoking in bed, drops his cigarette on the sheets, and starts a smoldering fire. The smoker dies of smoke inhalation; the majority of burns on the body occur after death. If the ME finds soot below the victim's larynx, esophagus, or stomach it implies the soot was swallowed and the victim was alive when the fire started.

Drug users also occasionally start accidental fires. On June 1, 1980, comedian Richard Pryor was badly burned when he tried to freebase cocaine (burning the drug in order to inhale the fumes). Freebasing involves the dangerous use of flammable solvents, including diethyl ether.

Smoke inhalation causes death in many fires, but people also die of burns or thermal injury during the fire or a few days after the event. Often when people die following a fire, it's because of fluid loss, shock, or respiratory failure due to damage caused by the inhalation of gases. Later deaths are often caused by sepsis or respiratory problems (DiMaio and DiMaio 2001).

Burn injuries range in four levels of severity, from first degree to fourth degree. First-degree burns are common, minor injuries with damage confined to the outer layer of skin (the epidermis). The burned area is initially red and swollen, but in live people, the damaged skin soon peels away to reveal fresh new skin. Sunburn is an example of a first-degree burn.

In a second-degree burn, the upper layers of the epidermis are damaged, producing blisters; this often happens in an injury caused by a hot liquid. Layers of the epidermis and the dermis are destroyed, and there may be some charring or blackening of the skin when the person suffers a third-degree burn; a survivor will need skin grafts. Electric shock can also create this kind of injury. A victim suffers charring of the epidermis, dermis, and underlying tissues in fourth-degree burns. On January 27, 1967, at Cape Kennedy, Florida, astronauts Roger Chaffee, Gus Grissom, and Edward

White died in a fire, their bodies charred, in an Apollo spacecraft mounted on a Saturn rocket (Grissom 1967).

Besides smoke and flame, heat can have a devastating impact on a body. The higher the fire's temperature, the greater the pressure within the person's skull. The skull is, after all, essentially a sealed vessel that contains fluid and brain tissue. As the heat increases, fluid and brain tissue may reach the boiling point, creating pressure that can burst the skull into numerous pieces. If during a homicide, however, a victim was shot in the head before the fire took hold, the hole in the skull would allow the pressure to vent. The more intact the skull, the easier it is for a forensic anthropologist to help identify the body (Bass and Jefferson 2003).

After enduring high temperatures, unburned skin may resemble seared leather. Burned bone will appear grayish white with heat fractures; it may be weak and brittle, and crumble when touched. Skin and flesh on the face may be burned away, exposing a heat-fractured skull. The hands and feet of badly burned bodies often disintegrate.

Body positioning can reveal clues to a person's death in a fire. In fires in a variety of settings, from houses and apartments to department stores and nightclubs, medical examiners commonly find decedents who exhibit a pugilistic attitude—a pose with hands raised and forward, fists clenched like a boxer's. Heat causes muscle fibers to coagulate, contract, and bend the limbs. If a fire victim was found lying on his side with his hands extended behind his back, he could be a homicide victim who was tied up. In research associated with the Institute of Forensic Medicine at the University of Freiburg, Germany, un-dissected bodies undergoing cremation showed a pugilistic attitude after approximately ten minutes at temperatures between 670 and 810 degrees Centigrade (Bohnert, Rost, and Pollak 1998; Miletich 2003).

Suicide by fire—also called self-immolation—is highly unusual, but when this occurs the victim typically pours a flammable liquid such as gasoline on her clothes and uses a match or lighter to set herself on fire. Not all people who set themselves on fire die right away. Some will die from complications later. Burn patterns may indicate if this person was standing, sitting, or lying when she ignited her clothes. Investigators should check her lighter or matches for fingerprints and take samples of clothing to test for the flammable liquid.

Homicide by fire, like suicide by fire, is also rare, although a perpetrator may start a fire to conceal a murder. But it's very difficult to completely burn up a body, as human tissue has high water content. So while the body may be very damaged on the surface, its insides are still identifiable. Arsonists may kill people unintentionally when they burn down a building (Barillo and Goode 1996; Pounder 1992).

When someone has died in a fire, it can be difficult for the medical examiner to differentiate between acute antemortem and postmortem burns because the body usually will not have survived long enough to show an inflammatory response—something that may not happen until a few days after the fire (DiMaio and DiMaio 2001). Blisters can develop postmortem as well.

If a burn victim is charred beyond recognition, the first thing an ME may do is order a complete X-ray of the body. This way the medical examiner can determine if there are any bullets or other significant details she needs to know. If fingerprints can't be taken, the ME will likely try to identify the person through dental records. The medical examiner may remove the victim's jaws to get the best image. A body this badly burned will not be viewed at the funeral, so this should not cause any problems with relatives.

Scalding burns, including steam, immersion, and splash burns, do not char or singe tissue like flame burns, but can be very damaging nevertheless. In an immersion burn, the medical examiner will see a clear line of demarcation between burned and unburned tissue. This type of burn can be seen on an infant who was bathed in too-hot water—a common form of child abuse. A splash burn is characterized by an irregular line over isolated areas of burned skin, usually round or oval in shape and caused by droplets of hot liquid. A steam burn can inflict serious, scald-like injuries and can kill a person if enough is inhaled into the air passages (Smock 2000).

The chances of being struck by lightning are slim indeed, but it does happen. A person who was struck by lightning and died may have Lichtenberg figures over his back, shoulders, buttocks, or legs. These rare marks are painless, red, fern-like or arboresque patterns. Lichtenberg figures tend to fade over a couple of days and do not leave behind scars or any discoloration, as would thermal or electrical burns. Biopsy specimens do not reveal pathological changes in epidermis, dermis, or collagen. German physicist Georg Christoph Lichtenberg first described Lichtenberg figures in 1777.

One cause of death that is not well understood is Sudden Infant Death Syndrome (SIDS), the abrupt and unexpected death of an infant aged one or younger. Even after a thorough autopsy, death scene investigation, and infant medical history review, these deaths are unexplainable. SIDS is also known as crib death or cot death.

The National SIDS Foundation first named this mysterious illness in 1962, and the SIDS Act was passed in 1974 to promote research and education. This syndrome usually occurs in apparently healthy infants and is associated with sleep; infants who sleep on their stomachs are more likely to die of SIDS than infants who sleep on their backs. These deaths occur almost always between 10 P.M. and 10 A.M., and more cases of SIDS are reported in fall and winter than in spring and summer. One clue is that respiratory infections are common among these infants prior to their death. A pink froth from the lungs sometimes foams around the infant's mouth after death from SIDS.

SIDS is also associated with a harmful prenatal environment: a mother younger than age twenty at the time of her first pregnancy who abused drugs and smoked cigarettes while pregnant, and who had a history of urinary tract infection or sexually transmitted disease. Three male infants die for every two female infants. Thousands of babies die from SIDS annually in the U.S., and police and the medical examiner must, by law, investigate every case.

If the death occurred in the infant's crib at home, police should note if the mattress was suitable for the size of the crib. A baby can become wedged between a mattress and the sides of the crib and suffocate. If the death occurred in an adult-size bed, officers should find out if one or more people were sleeping with the infant and if they were impaired by alcohol or drugs. Police should also be alert for other dangers to babies in the immediate surroundings, such as the proximity of toys in relation to the infant, use of a vaporizer, state of cleanliness of the surroundings, and any pets capable of suffocating the infant.

It may sound like an urban myth or an old wives' tale, but cases of cats smothering babies have been recorded. In 1995 in New Zealand, a twenty-four-day-old baby boy was found dead in his crib, an adult cat lying on his face. An autopsy excluded disease as the cause of death, but cat fur was found in the baby's mouth and larynx, as well as conjunctival petechiae (tiny red or purple hemorrhages in the inner membranes of the eyelids) in his eyes. The coroner accepted that the cat suffocated the infant (Bignall 1995; Kearney, Dahl, and Stalsberg 1982).

In investigating a case of SIDS, the medical examiner will be especially attentive to the infant's clothes, formula, over-the-counter or prescribed drugs, body temperature, rigor mortis, postmortem lividity (PML), and body fluids: vomit, blood, or mucus. The infant's medical history records and interviews with parents or guardians can provide the police and the ME with information about the infant's health condition prior to his death. Some questions to ask include whether the infant ever required oxygen, a pacemaker, or an apnea monitor; had food intolerances; or had to be taken to a hospital emergency room. At autopsy the bladder of a SIDS victim is almost always empty, and usually there are petechial hemorrhages on the lungs, heart, and thymus (an organ of the developing immune system located behind the breastbone). An infant with facial and external upper chest petechiae (small hemorrhages), however, did not die of SIDS (Berry 1992; Bignall 1995; Byard and Krous 1999; Havill 2001; Lundstrom and Sharpe 1991; Weyand 2004).

Petechiae can be a significant clue in a death investigation. Someone who died from asphyxia will have petechiae in a number of places, including the lining of the lower eyelids, around the lips, and inside the cheeks. Sometimes linear hemorrhages are mistaken for petechiae, however. Linear hemorrhages occur at the time of death or after, but are not associated with a specific disease or injury. A linear hemorrhage may be approximately a millimeter in width and a quarter of an inch in length (Wecht, Saitz, and Curriden 2003).

One of the critical conditions for human life is adequate access to oxygen. But a person doesn't have to drown or be strangled in order to asphyxiate. Sometimes a lack of cooperation with the law causes the trouble—or at least sets in motion a chain of events that can lead to death by asphyxiation.

In the course of their duties, police have the option to hog-tie a violent person in order to get him under control. The method is to bind the person's hands and feet together behind his back and place the person on his stomach. This position is physically incapacitating and makes breathing difficult—so difficult that a hog-tied person could die. If this happens, a medical examiner would generally attribute the death to positional asphyxia: the inability of the person to breathe because of his body position. This leads to oxygen deficiency in the blood, which disturbs the body's chemistry and heart rhythm and causes a fatal heart attack. Although hypoxia can occur in minutes, it can occur more quickly if the person who has been behaving aggressively is already out of breath.

A hog-tied person with a large abdomen has a higher risk of dying of positional asphyxia because lying on one's belly forces the contents of the abdomen upward. This puts pressure on the diaphragm, a muscle critical for respiration, and restricts its movement. A person who is psychotic because of drugs or alcohol is also at high risk of death from positional asphyxia, as he may be experiencing intoxicant-induced vigorous muscular activity. This person can lose his breath quickly and may have difficulty recovering; oxygen deficiency and heart rhythm irregularity, and then possibly death, may follow. At autopsy, the forensic pathologist sometimes sees signs of heart attack or stroke (Parent 2006; Reay 1996).

Other forms of asphyxia are more intentional, such as in "burking." In this type of murder, the perpetrator suffocates the victim and leaves few or no indications of violence on the body. Burking gets its name from two men who were on trial for the sixteen West Port Murders in Edinburgh, Scotland, in 1829: William Burke (1792–1829) and William Hare (?–c. 1860). Burke and Hare, born in Ireland, arrived in Edinburgh around 1818 to work on construction of the Union Canal. They heard about grave robbing and the selling of bodies to doctors, who needed corpses for anatomy classes. So Burke and Hare apparently robbed graves and sold the corpses to Dr. Robert Knox (1791–1862), who taught anatomy at Edinburgh University. Burke would later deny that he and Hare ever robbed graves.

However, the men lured victims to the lodging house where they lived, plied the victims with liquor, and "burked" them. While one perpetrator put a hand over the nose and mouth of the victim, the other perpetrator sat on the victim's chest and prevented him from breathing. Knox's students became suspicious about the number of bodies he had for dissection, at a time when it was difficult to obtain bodies. Police also became suspicious about the disappearance of a number of people, and a police investigation led to Burke and Hare. Burke was hanged on January 28, 1829, and his body dissected in public. A wallet made from his tanned skin is at the Anatomy Museum of the Royal College of Surgeons in Edinburgh. Hare gave evidence against Burke in exchange for immunity; he hurriedly left Edinburgh after police released him in early February 1829. Knox was not charged with a crime, but his career waned and he eventually left Edinburgh for London, where he had a position at the Cancer Hospital (Baden and Roach 2001; Burke 2004; MacGowan 2004).

In 1998, in Las Vegas, Nevada, a casino executive died in a way that some people claimed was murder by burking. This case is another example of how respected experts can disagree on critical issues.

At 3:55 P.M. on September 17, twenty-six-year-old Sandy Murphy, the live-in girlfriend of Ted Binion, fifty-five, frantically told a Las Vegas Metropolitan Police Department (LVMPD) 911 operator that Binion was not breathing. She led paramedics to a den in the house on Palomino Lane. Binion was lying face up on a sleeping mat, hands at his sides, feet straight out, a comforter partially covering his lower body. His skin was gray. Paramedic Steven Reincke determined that Binion did not have a pulse, his body was cold to the touch, and his jaw was stiff with rigor mortis. Reincke believed Binion had been dead for at least two hours. Binion was wearing underwear and a dress shirt, the shirt pushed up on his chest.

Nearby on the carpet was an empty prescription bottle for the antianxiety drug Xanax. According to information on the bottle, Dr. Enrique Lacayo, Binion's neighbor, prescribed the Xanax on September 16, the previous day. Three disposable lighters, an open pack of cigarettes, and a remote control for a TV or VCR also lay nearby on the carpet. There was no suicide note and no obvious signs of foul play, but there was a slight abrasion on the back of Binion's right hand, an abrasion on the front of his left knee, and a reddish mark approximately in the center of his chest.

In the bathroom adjacent to the den, investigators found a pocketknife with brownish residue on the blade, an ashtray, and a clean piece of foil. They found several pieces of crumpled foil and a piece of pink rubber balloon in the bathroom trash can. A piece of red balloon was on the floor. Binion's drug dealer had delivered twelve balloons of black tar heroin to Binion on the previous day. The casino executive had "chased the dragon"—heated heroin on tinfoil and then inhaled the smoke. This is the least effective way to use heroin—and least dangerous—compared to injecting it with a needle or administering it with a suppository. Apparently no one has ever died from heroin by chasing the dragon.

Between 1987 and 1997, Binion's problems ranged from an arrest for heroin trafficking to suspensions of his gaming license. The Nevada Casino Gaming Control Board believed he had connections with alleged underworld figures and, in March 1998, permanently revoked his gaming license.

Murphy, who appeared to be extremely upset at the death scene, was taken by ambulance to nearby Valley Hospital. At 5:29 P.M., Dr. Brian

Kominsky examined her; another doctor prescribed Valium, which she refused to take when nurse Larry Krev tried to administer it. Approximately twenty minutes later, Murphy had calmed down considerably without Valium. Krev believed her behavior was theatrical, and mentioned this to a detective at the hospital.

At Binion's residence, lead investigator Detective James Buczek and other LVPD detectives studied the death scene. Usually in a drug-overdose death, investigators see a significant amount of vomit. In this case, they saw traces of vomit in the immediate area of Binion's body. Also, the position of the body made them suspicious: it looked as if it were laid out at a funeral home. Buczek suspected someone had cleaned Binion's body and the death scene before police were contacted. It looked as though the death scene had been staged.

Dr. Larry Simms, chief medical examiner of Clark County, arrived at the scene. As Simms entered the den from the dining room, he noted several dried droplets of a fluid that looked like gastric content, its pattern linear and ending where Binion's body was located when paramedics arrived. This suggested that Binion's body was moved. While conducting Binion's autopsy on September 18, Simms noted livor mortis on Binion's right arm and the right side of his face and back—indicating he was lying on his right side, not his back, when livor was fixed after death (see Chapter 2 for more on livor mortis). Simms also noted a circular "erosion," about half an inch in diameter, in the center of Binion's chest. Simms suggested that shirt buttons could have been pressed into Binion's chest during a struggle, likely producing the erosion. The autopsy revealed a drug overdose was the cause of death, with the following drugs in Binion's system: morphine, a breakdown product of heroin; Xanax (alprazolam); and Valium (diazepam). Binion either ate or snorted the heroin and Xanax. Witnesses said he was not known to snort drugs or ingest heroin orally. His sister, Becky Behnen, did not believe that Binion committed suicide.

On September 19, two days after Binion's death, Nye County Sheriff's Department Sergeant Ed Howard and Deputy Dean Pennock were dispatched to check on Binion's underground vault in Pahramp, Nevada, after a report of a disturbance at the site. The officers found Rick Tabish and two other men, David Mattsen and Michael Milot, with Milot operating an excavator. They had about twenty-four tons of Binion's silver—at some estimates worth 7 million dollars—inside a tractor-trailer nearby. Tabish said he was removing the silver to sell it, so he could give the proceeds to Binion's teenage daughter, Bonnie. Police arrested Tabish, Mattsen, and Milot on numerous charges, including burglary and grand larceny (Kenworthy 1998; Macy 1999; O'Connell 2000).

On October 2, Simms listed alprazolam (also known by the trade name Xanax) and opiate intoxication as the cause of death on Binion's death certificate. The manner of death was "pending police investigation." Authorities continued to investigate Binion's death. Meanwhile, Tom Dillard, a private investigator, investigated on behalf of the Binion family.

On March 15, 1999, nearly six months after the death, Clark County Coroner Ron Flud changed the manner of death from undetermined to homicide. Police sources suggested Flud made the change because investigators suspected the death scene was staged, while numerous people said they believed Murphy and Tabish killed Binion. About three months later, on June 24, 1999, police arrested Sandy Murphy and Rick Tabish on charges of murder, conspiracy, and robbery at a supermarket in Las Vegas. Police contended that interviews, phone records, and medical evidence supported their claim that Murphy and Tabish, secret lovers, murdered Binion to get some of his fortune. Binion had been suspicious of Murphy, particularly of her involvement with Tabish, and had changed his will a day prior to his death.

The prosecution alleged that Murphy and Tabish smothered Binion with a pillow or a hand. Forensic pathologists with opposing views testified. Dr. Michael Baden, forensic pathologist and former chief medical examiner for New York City, testified for the prosecution and claimed Binion died of forced suffocation. He said an obstruction had blocked Binion's nose and mouth and that pressure had been exerted on his chest. Baden said the manner of death was "pending police investigation," as drug levels were too low to have caused death. In drug overdose deaths, forensic pathologists see froth coming up the decedent's windpipe and through the nose and mouth, but this was not seen in Binion's death. Various bruises could have appeared shortly before or shortly after death. Baden noted that skin was rubbed off around Binion's mouth and nose. Baden also pointed to the capillaries that had burst in Binion's eyes, saying this happened during an increase in blood pressure in the face. Forced suffocation, in his view, produced this pressure.

Dr. Cyril Wecht, forensic pathologist and coroner of Allegheny County, Pennsylvania, was brought forward by the defense. Wecht's opinion was that Binion died of a drug overdose. Unlike Baden, Wecht did not see petechial hemorrhaging in photographs of Binion's eyes; this type of hemorrhaging, characterized by red dots the size of a pin's head, indicates sudden oxygen deprivation or a significant rise in blood pressure. Wecht said the redness around Binion's mouth resembled the facial redness some men have after shaving.

Wecht said he would have expected to find trauma to Binion's external neck or trachea if the casino exec had been strangled or suffocated. He added that if Binion had been burked, the autopsy would have revealed blue-hued congestion in his head from blood low in oxygen trapped above the lungs because of the pressure on his chest. He saw no signs of struggle and no defense wounds consistent with suffocation. Although individually none of the drugs constituted a lethal dose, in Wecht's opinion the mix of drugs collectively was lethal. Wecht said that Binion died of an overdose, that suicide was the manner of death, and that drug overdose was the mechanism of death.

On May 19, 2000, after deliberating for eight days, a jury at the Clark County Courthouse in Las Vegas found Murphy and Tabish guilty on all counts. On September 15, 2000, Judge Joseph T. Bonaventure sentenced Murphy and Tabish to life in prison with the possibility of parole. However, on July 14, 2003, the Nevada Supreme Court ordered a new trial for the defendants because errors by Judge Bonaventure prejudiced jurors against the defendants. The pair were acquitted at the second trial; however, both face one to five years of prison time for stealing Binion's silver collection (Baden and Roach 2001; German 2001; King 2001; Wecht, Saitz, and Curriden 2003).

A drowning person also struggles with a lack of oxygen, but the death process differs. Let's look at an example of a woman drowning in a river. While she fights to survive, her body will be in an almost vertical position, her head tilted back, face turned up, arms thrashing at the water's surface, with little leg movement. As she tires and sinks below the water line, at some point she will gasp for air—it is a reflex. Water then enters her mouth; the epiglottis (a flap of cartilage at the root of the tongue) closes over her airway. Breathing becomes impossible for a time. Without oxygen, she will soon become unconscious and experience respiratory arrest. The amount of air in her lungs and her body weight determine how soon she sinks to the river bottom. Her heart no longer pumps blood, her vital organs no longer receive oxygen-rich blood, and her skin turns blue due to a lack of oxygen. Death occurs within minutes. Later, gases form and build up in her intestinal tract, and her abdomen bloats. Gradually, her body rises to the surface where it floats, her head in a facedown position.

Once she's taken from the water, rescuers see a white froth or foam bubbling from her mouth and nostrils. This foam is made of water, air, and mucus and can indicate the drowning victim was alive when she submerged. Sometimes the froth is tinged with blood and is pinkish in color. Not every decedent with froth on the mouth drowned, however. Some people who die of heart disease or drug overdose have froth, and some drowning victims have no froth. In our example, as the medical examiner wipes the foam away, pressure on the victim's chest wall causes more foam to exude from her nostrils and mouth. This foam is also present in the trachea and main air passages. The ME notes river sediment on the victim's clothes; this confirms the body was at the bottom of the river.

During his death investigation, the ME is alert for any clues that reveal how the woman died—if she drowned or died some other way; if she drowned where she was found; if any signs point to foul play; or if her death was accidental or a suicide. Branches or other objects in her hand, due to cadaveric spasm, indicate the victim was alive and conscious when she submerged. Victims who strive to survive often have bruised or ruptured muscles, particularly of the neck and chest. After the drowning victim is taken to the ME's office and placed overnight in a cooler, decomposition advances because bacteria from her lungs and intestines move throughout her vascular system. At autopsy, the ME may find evidence of bleeding in the sinuses, as the victim's attempts to breathe during drowning subjected the sinuses to significant pressure. A large quantity of water and debris, such as silt or weeds, in her stomach suggests she was alive when she entered the water. The absence of water in the stomach suggests that the drowning victim either died rapidly or was dead before submersion. Comparing debris and chemicals recovered from her stomach and lungs with a sample of water where her body was found will confirm if she did indeed drown in that location. But even though her stomach may contain silt or weeds, that is not necessarily proof of drowning.

The lungs are sometimes waterlogged and sometimes overinflated. There is a physiological difference between a person who drowns in fresh water and a person who drowns in seawater. Fresh water rapidly enters the lungs and then the circulatory system; blood volume increases and produces strain on the heart. This blood dilution alters blood chemistry and red blood cells break down. Seawater, on the other hand, draws fluid from blood plasma into the lungs. This does not increase the strain on the heart. For this reason, people who are drowning tend to survive longer in salt water than in fresh water (Becker 2005; Lerner and Lerner 2006; Pounder 1992; Temple 2005).

One high-profile drowning case in the late 1960s created great public controversy medically and legally, especially as it involved a powerful married politician and his young female employee. Part of the doubt and debate that lingered in this case was due to the fact that a medical examiner without forensic pathology training made key decisions—including the decision that a quick external exam was all that was needed in this particular death investigation. Sometime between 11:15 P.M. on Friday, July 18, 1969, and 1 A.M. on Saturday, July 19, an Oldsmobile with two occupants drove off Dike Bridge and plunged into the depths of Poucha Pond on Chappaquiddick Island, Massachusetts. Thirty-seven-year-old Massachusetts Senator Ted Kennedy was at the wheel; his twenty-eight-year-old secretary, Mary Jo Kopechne, sat beside him. Earlier, Kennedy and eleven other people, including Kennedy's cousin Joe Gargan and Paul Markham, a former U.S. attorney, had attended a party in a rented cottage on the island. The guests included six unmarried girls who had worked on Robert Kennedy's campaign, as well as six married men.

Kopechne drowned in the submerged car. Kennedy, who escaped, later said he had attempted to rescue Kopechne but was unsuccessful; the water was dark and had a fast-moving current. Yet he waited ten hours before notifying police. Instead, he returned to his hotel room. When he eventually called police, he spoke to the police chief of Edgartown, Dominick James Arena, on July 19, explaining it took him time to fully realize what had happened. Kennedy told Arena that on the previous day, Friday, at

approximately 11:15 P.M., he was driving to the ferry landing at Chappaquiddick when he took a wrong turn and drove off the bridge.

After talking to Kennedy, Chief Arena unsuccessfully tried to enter the submerged car. Later, scuba diver John N. Farrar examined the upside-down car
and saw that the ignition was on, the car was in drive, the brake was off, the
light switch was on, and the gas tank was full. The window on the driver's side
was down, and the driver's door was locked. Farrar also noted that Kopechne's
body was in the uppermost part of the upside-down footwell of the automobile.
Her arms were bent at right angles, her hands tightly gripping the edge of the
back seat. This position let her hold her head up, straining upward toward an
air pocket. Farrar maneuvered her body through a window of the car; she
floated to the surface. As a tow truck operator turned the car over and pulled it
to shore, air trapped inside bubbled from the car. At about 9:15 A.M. on Saturday, Associate Medical Examiner Dr. Donald R. Mills arrived to examine Mary
Jo Kopechne, who had been submerged eight or nine hours. Mills was a general
practitioner with no training in forensic pathology.

Kopechne's body, on a stretcher and covered by a blue blanket, was in full
rigor mortis. Her arms were stretched outward from the shoulders as if to
ward off a blow, hands in a semi-claw position. There was white froth about
the nose and mouth and traces of blood trickling from the left nostril. Mills
examined her skull, throat, and neck, and found no fractures. He could not
hear any sound when he placed a stethoscope over the heart. When he
tapped her chest, water welled up from inside her lungs and came out of
her mouth and nose. Mills did not see any trauma to her back or abdomen.
Her uterus did not appear to be enlarged; she probably was not pregnant.
He concluded drowning was the cause of death and that an autopsy was not
needed, although it was an option that he as well as Edmund S. Dinis, the
district attorney for the Southern District of Massachusetts, could exercise.
Mills's examination had lasted about eight or nine minutes.

Dr. Mills released the body to Eugene Frieh, an undertaker who had
attended the death scene. Mills emphasized that the body was not to be
embalmed until the ME had consulted with the district attorney's office and
the state police regarding his decision about an autopsy.

Mills rode with Frieh in the hearse that took Kopechne's body to the funeral home at Vineyard Haven. Frieh and his assistant undressed her in the
preparation room. A blood sample was taken from her left armpit. They put
a body block under her diaphragm; abdominal compression yielded less
than a teacup of moisture and pinkish froth. Frieh was surprised; he
expected more moisture and froth. Usually a person who drowns has consumed quarts or gallons of water. Frieh wondered if Kopechne had suffocated to death rather than drowned. During his career, he had embalmed
twenty-four drowning victims; each had been full of water. But Frieh did
not see any bruises or marks on her body except for a slight abrasion on
the knuckle of her left hand. So Frieh delayed embalming Kopechne,

believing that Mills would want an autopsy after all. Later, however, Mills signed a filled-out death certificate brought to him by Dun Gifford, a legislative assistant to Kennedy. The cause of death on the certificate was asphyxiation by immersion in an overturned and submerged automobile.

Farrar, the scuba diver, and Frieh, the mortician, agreed that Kopechne did not drown; they believed she had suffocated by inhaling her expelled carbon dioxide after the air pocket emptied. A person who drowns sinks for seventy-two to one hundred hours before their body becomes buoyant. Kopechne's body had not sunk to the bottom of the inside of the car; it was at the inside top. Farrar, who believed she had enough oxygen to survive for three or four hours, thought she could have been rescued if help had been called immediately after the accident. According to Farrar, he could have been at the location in twenty-five minutes.

Rumors began circulating that Kennedy and Kopechne had engaged in immoral behavior before the accident and that Kopechne was pregnant. The blood sample taken from Kopechne was analyzed by state police and revealed a blood alcohol content of 0.09 percent, indicating she was not legally drunk when she died, nor were there any barbiturates in her body.

On Sunday morning, July 20, twenty-four hours after Kopechne's death, district attorney Dinis requested an autopsy be performed before her body was taken off Chappaquiddick. He was concerned about drowning versus suffocation as the cause of death, as well as about inconsistencies in statements Kennedy made to police about rescue efforts. Lieutenant George Killen, Dinis's chief investigator, told him that her body had been embalmed and flown to Pennsylvania by people acting on behalf of Kennedy. Massachusetts officials would have no legal authority over the body after it was in Pennsylvania. According to Massachusetts law, the medical cause of death could be changed only after an autopsy.

Mary Jo Kopechne was buried on July 22 in Plymouth, Pennsylvania. If it could be proven that Kennedy abandoned Kopechne while she was alive and breathing, that he did not notify police and rescue personnel at that time, and that this contributed to her death, then he was guilty of manslaughter. Legal activity extended into January 1970 as two opposing groups battled. One side, including district attorney Dinis, forensic pathology expert witnesses, and other supporters, doubted that drowning was the cause of Kopechne's death and were skeptical about Kennedy's account of events. Other causes of death could not be excluded on the basis of only an external examination. The other side, comprising attorneys, forensic pathology expert witnesses, and supporters of Kennedy, argued that exhuming Kopechne's body for an autopsy would not change the fact that drowning was the cause of death, even if physical injuries were found that had been overlooked prior to embalming and burial. Both groups were aware that judicial decisions to follow would impact the political future of a man who could become a U.S. president.

On July 31, district attorney Dinis requested an inquest into the death. His purpose was to determine if Kopechne had died from an act of negligence by anyone other than herself. On September 18, Dinis, in a Petition for Exhumation and Autopsy in the Court of Common Pleas for Luzerne County, Pennsylvania, claimed that blood was seen in Mary Jo Kopechne's mouth and nose. An incident prior to the Dike Bridge accident, possibly an earlier accident, might account for the presence of this blood. She also had blood on the back of her blouse. On September 24, Cardinal Richard Cushing, one of the most eminent religious figures in the U.S. and a longtime close friend of the Kennedys, spoke to Kopechne's parents in Wilkes-Barre. He told them that, as Christians, they should oppose the exhumation of their daughter's body for the purpose of an autopsy. The parents subsequently filed a petition to bar the autopsy.

On December 8, just after he was reelected in Wilkes-Barre, Pennsylvania, Judge Bernard C. Brominski denied the exhumation and autopsy petition. His reason: the facts presented were insufficient to support a finding for cause of death other than asphyxiation by immersion.

Later, between January 5 and January 8, 1970, Kennedy and twenty-six other witnesses testified at Judge James Boyle's secret inquest in Edgartown. In his final report regarding the inquest, Judge Boyle said there was no evidence that any air remained in the car after it was immersed.

In spite of the scandal, public relations issues, and legal battles, Kennedy did not resign as senator. But in 1980 Kennedy lost the bid for the presidency to Jimmy Carter (Damore 1988; Kappel 1989).

While the dangers in one's environment are not always controllable—particularly if one is riding in the passenger seat of a sinking car—medical examiners can improve safety in their communities by drawing public attention to hazards and advocating for change at the legislative level. And that can create a great deal of job satisfaction.

In the next chapter, we look at dangers some people engage in willingly— at least at first: illegal drugs.

5

DEATH AND DRUGS

IT'S A BIT ironic that controlled substance laws have never been stricter than they are today, yet the availability and variety of street drugs continue to grow. And as a consequence, so does the number of dead addicts on a medical examiner's to-do list. As new "designer drugs" appear on the scene, medical examiners are often some of the first to know.

In 1970, efforts to coordinate drug laws manifested in the Controlled Substances Act (CSA), which consolidated laws about the possession, sale, or manufacture of drugs and other substances. These drugs and substances are classified into five categories (Schedules I to V) according to their potential for abuse. A drug taken internally for a non-medical reason is a drug that is abused. Although the CSA is federal legislation, states may add other drugs and substances to deal with state issues. Drugs allocated to one schedule may be allocated to another schedule, depending on ongoing research results.

Schedule I drugs have a high potential for abuse and include heroin and LSD. These drugs, with the exception of marijuana, for example, are thought of as having no medical use. However, medical research regarding marijuana has been allowed in some states.

Schedule II drugs have a high potential for abuse but have some medical use. These include cocaine and morphine. The potential for abuse decreases again for Schedule III drugs; these include anabolic steroids and some barbiturates, drugs that also have some medical use. Schedule IV drugs such as Talwin and Valium have a low potential for abuse and have accepted medical use. Schedule V drugs have a low potential for abuse, have medical use, and include cough suppressant that contains codeine (Houde 1999).

Regardless of their classification, illegal drugs are used widely. In 2002, approximately 2 million Americans were using cocaine; 567,000 of them were using crack cocaine, a form of purified cocaine. Also at this time, approximately 166,000 persons were using heroin. Of course, some of these users became medical examiner cases (Aschenbrenner and Venable 2006).

We'll look at how that happens in this chapter. Some of the usual suspects include the aforementioned heroin, cocaine, and LSD, but also the new kids on the block: cherry meth, ecstasy, and ketamine, referred to as "designer drugs." These will be discussed in more detail later in the text.

Heroin, an extract of opium from poppies, is a white crystalline odorless powder that has a bitter taste. This drug produces euphoria and has an analgesic effect on individuals who use it, but the addict can never fully repeat his first high. In fact, although he tries by increasing his heroin dose, he will have more and more difficulty attaining the euphoria he initially experienced. Depression, drowsiness, inability to concentrate, decreased appetite, constipation, and decreased libido are also associated with heroin use. Anxiety, insomnia, nausea, and vomiting are part of withdrawal.

"Smack," "horse," and "scag" are examples of heroin's street names. Dealers "cut" (add to) heroin with one or more substances, including soap powder, sugar, and talcum powder, in order to extend the inventory and make more money. Some substances can change the color of white heroin to dark brown or black. By the time addicts buy heroin on the street, the potency of the heroin has been drastically decreased.

Heroin addicts get their fix by inhalation ("snorting"), injecting under the skin ("skin popping"), and intravenous injection (into a vein or "mainlining"). The addict who mainlines sprinkles the heroin onto a spoon, bottle cap, or can, adds water, and then heats the mixture over a flame. She draws the heroin into a syringe and injects it, usually into a vein in the forearm. Within seconds, the body changes injected heroin into morphine that binds to pain-suppressing receptors in the brain that also produce euphoria. After a vein becomes hardened or clogged, due to additives used to cut the heroin, the addict uses another vein. Eventually, the addict injects the drug into the feet, between toes, or into the thighs or stomach.

Another method of inhaling heroin is "chasing the dragon," also referred to as "chui lung," "Chinesing," and "Chinese blowing." What's required: powdered heroin, base powder, tinfoil (approximately the size found in a package of cigarettes), a lighter, and a paper tube (similar to a drinking straw). The smoker uses a metal instrument to smooth out the foil until the foil is highly polished. Then he or she folds the foil in half and places the heroin and base powder about half an inch apart in the crease. The smoker places the flame of the lighter to the foil underneath the base powder, which liquefies and mixes with the heroin. He or she simultaneously tilts the foil back and forth, and directs the paper tube, held in the mouth, over the foil, inhaling the vapor emanating from the heated mixture. To experience the maximum effect of the vapor, the smoker uses the paper tube to "chase" the "smoky tail" of the sticky liquid, which moves back and forth ("wriggles like a Chinese dragon") in the crease of the foil until a black stain is the only thing remaining.

Heroin smoking originated in Shanghai in the 1920s, spread across Eastern Asia, and then spread to the U.S. over the next decade. Chasing the dragon originated in or near Hong Kong in the 1950s.

British chemist C.R. Alder Wright first developed heroin in 1874, when he boiled morphine with acetic anhydride and made diacetylmorphine, otherwise known as heroin. Heroin, like morphine and codeine before it, became an ingredient of patent medicines and was available in pharmacies in powder form. Some injected themselves with it, overdosed, and died. In 1898, Bayer and Company, the German chemical-pharmaceutical firm, introduced heroin as a cough suppressant. Bayer scientist Heinrich Dreser was seeking a substitute for morphine, as morphine was addictive, and believed that heroin was the answer. So heroin not only substituted for morphine but became a treatment for tuberculosis, pneumonia, and other ailments. The opinion of the day continued to be that heroin was not addictive.

Although signs became commonplace in the 1890s that heroin might be dangerous, it was not until 1916 that Public Health Service Hospitals in the U.S. finally heeded the warnings and discontinued dispensing the drug. In 1920, the American Medical Association (AMA) adopted a resolution that opposed the importation, manufacture, sale, or use of heroin. However, by the 1920s, heroin misuse was common in the American underworld, with a minimum of 10,000 heroin-dependent individuals using 76,000 ounces annually in New York.

Heroin in twenty-first-century New York is available in 3/4-inch by 1 1/2-inch glassine envelopes, sealed with transparent tape. Sometimes these envelopes are folded in thirds horizontally and are sold in colored plastic bags, which prevent the heroin from dissolving if the addict puts the bag into his or her mouth or if the bag gets wet. This heroin has a "brand name," including "Elevator," "Silver Bullet," and "Back-draft," stamped on each envelope. Each brand sells at a specific location known as a "spot." Addicts use brand names to judge the quality of heroin. The greater the quality, the better the euphoria (Fernandez 1998; Green and Levy 1976; Marlowe 1999).

Although the person who "chases the dragon" avoids the HIV and hepatitis infections associated with injecting heroin with shared needles, health risks include a brain disease called spongiform leukoencephalopathy. On the autopsy table, the medical examiner will see the white matter of the addict's brain covered with microscopic spongelike, fluid-filled spaces. The disease affects specific cells and causes them to block nerve impulses in the brain. Some heroin smokers become uncoordinated and have difficulty moving and talking because the cerebellum and motor pathways are the areas of the brain most severely affected. The estimated mortality rate of spongiform leukoencephalopathy is 23 percent (Chasing 2004; Chasing the Dragon 1999; Hill, Cooper, and Perry 2000; The Smoking 2004; Strang, Griffiths, and Gossop 1997).

Cocaine, one of the oldest known drugs, is an alkaloid, a chemical that contains plant-produced nitrogen. Derived from the leaves of the coca bush,

Erythroxylon coca, cocaine is a powerful central nervous system stimulant and local anesthetic. Doctors use cocaine to anesthetize parts of a patient's nose, eyes, and ears during surgery.

In its mildest, fresh-off-the-bush form, the drug has helped indigenous people in South America manage long grueling hours of cultivating crops at high altitudes for thousands of years. As they worked the rough terrain, these hardy farmers would refresh their energy reserves by chewing some coca leaves. Coca bushes are also now cultivated in Peru and Bolivia.

Today, cocaine manufacturers make the drug by first temporarily storing the leaves in drums that contain kerosene or other solvent. The leaves process into a coffee-colored paste, which is then sold to illegal laboratories where the paste is refined into pure cocaine. This bitter, white, and odorless crystalline powder has been an abused substance for over a century.

Like heroin, cocaine was initially an uncontrolled substance that was used widely in medicinal preparations. In the early 1900s, after years of claims by patent-medicine quacks that cocaine could cure numerous ailments including fatigue, asthma, and stomach discomfort, the government became aware of the drug's addictive and psychologically debilitating nature. The Harrison Act of 1914 restricted access to cocaine to individuals with a doctor's prescription. Anyone who illegally distributed or sold cocaine was subject to fines and imprisonment.

Cocaine offers users a sense of euphoria as well as a near-manic energy and artificial confidence. But, like heroin, street cocaine usually contains a variety of additives such as powdered milk or talcum powder, or other stimulant drugs including procaine or lidocaine. These substances dilute the purity of the cocaine, and drug dealers make more money when they have more "cocaine" to sell.

Usually, cocaine is sniffed ("snorted") through a straw, after the cocaine powder is drawn out in narrow "lines," approximately one to two inches long. Cocaine is also injected under the skin or into a vein, or applied to mucous membranes or to the genitalia for absorption through the skin. When sniffed or injected, it rapidly produces a feeling of great energy and an increase in psychological alertness, as well as a reduction in hunger and thirst. The user's heart rate, respiration, body temperature, and perspiration increase. People high on cocaine believe they can do almost anything. Side effects include cocaine psychosis, characterized by hallucinations, paranoid delusions, and a tendency toward violent behavior. The person afflicted will have disturbing and tactile hallucinations; a common one is that white bugs are crawling under her skin. This perception, "Magnan's sign," derives its name from the French psychiatrist Valentin Jacques Joseph Magnan (1835–1916).

Medical examiners see a variety of the drug's deadly effects when they open up cocaine addicts during a death investigation. Cocaine users may die from cardiac arrest, convulsions, or depression of the respiratory or vasomotor centers. Located in the brain, the respiratory center integrates sensory information about blood levels of oxygen and carbon dioxide and determines how the respiratory muscles react to these levels. The brain's vasomotor center regulates the diameter of blood vessels. A constricted blood vessel can cause a stroke or disruption of the blood supply to the brain. If the disruption is not restored, the person will suffer permanent brain damage (Awareness 2004; Smart 1983; The Story 2004).

Cocaine is a vasoconstrictor—an agent that causes blood vessels to narrow—making this drug a very risky choice for those with heart disease. When a person sniffs the drug, this narrowing effect also includes blood vessels in the nose. Chronic sniffing deprives nasal tissues of blood, killing these tissues. Perforations and other damage are often seen in the nasal septum, the vertical plane of mucous membrane-covered cartilage and bone separating the nostrils. Blood vessels in the mucous membranes provide the cartilage with nutrition, but fewer nutrients are available when blood vessels are constricted. Furthermore, street cocaine has additives that usually act as chemical irritants, further damaging the mucous membranes.

A surgeon may treat septum perforation by devising a plastic button that precisely fits a perforation. A medical examiner who examines a dead person's nose and sees not only the button but also a loss of nasal hair may assume the person chronically sniffed cocaine, pending test results of the decedent's urine (Perforated 2004; Picture 2004; Villa 1999).

People with cocaine in their possession have attempted to hide the evidence by swallowing the drug when they see police approaching them. Often, police have been alerted by the drug user's suspicious behavior or have received a report that this person may be carrying drug paraphernalia. The results for the user can be deadly.

On October 25, 2003, airport screeners at Seattle-Tacoma International Airport in Washington State found a drug pipe in the carry-on luggage of Desseria B. Whitmore, a fifty-two-year-old Bank of America assistant vice president. Whitmore, who intended to fly to Spokane, twice tried to flee from police. She then swallowed a plastic bag of cocaine and began to suffocate. Paramedics were unable to revive her and a subsequent autopsy revealed that she died of acute cocaine intoxication and asphyxia at the airport (Rivera 2003).

Some people stash cocaine and other drugs in their bodies for a living. Called "body packers," they store the drugs in sealed condoms, balloons, plastic bags. or other soft, waterproof containers and swallow them or tuck them into their rectums or vaginas. Body packers, also referred to as "mules" or "swallowers," are known to travel by air from cocaine-producing countries such as Colombia—perhaps the biggest cocaine producer in the world—to big market countries such as the U.S. and Canada. A body packer who swallows drug packets typically uses laxatives or enemas to induce a bowel movement at his destination. In the 1990s, these smugglers tried to elude X ray detection by concealing drugs in machine-pressed pellets made from sealed latex glove fingers that were coated with wax and other materials, including transparent tape and carbon paper. Swallowers train for their work by pushing condoms filled with grapes down their throat. Some swallowers numb their throat—and gag reflex—with Chloraseptic (Taylor and Linedecker 1998).

All this becomes the business of medical examiners fairly often, as containers can break and empty their contents into the body packer's gastrointestinal tract. The smuggler's packaging may also leak or, if ill chosen, have a semi-permeable membrane, allowing cocaine to gradually be absorbed and overdose the carrier. Symptoms include mydriasis (excessive dilation of the pupil of the eye), seizures, acute toxic psychosis, and coma before death from acute cocaine toxicity.

Body packers may swallow as many as 100 packages without suffering ill consequences aboard aircraft or en route to or in hotel rooms in their destination countries. But some of these smugglers may end up with one or more packages lodged in their intestines, a potentially life-threatening problem (Sachs 2004; Wetli and Mittleman 1981; Yanai and Hiss 1999).

A highly addictive form of purified cocaine is crack cocaine, made from mixing cocaine and baking soda with water and then adding heat. The mixture is dried, broken into tiny chunks, and packaged by dealers into small vials for sale. Crack is usually smoked in glass pipes. The stem of one of these pipes is called "the devil's dick."

Crack produces euphoria by rapidly and intensely stimulating the part of the brain associated with emotions. The faster cocaine reaches the brain, the greater the euphoria experienced by the user. Inhaled crack cocaine vapor reaches the brain in less than fifteen seconds—much faster than snorting regular cocaine. The high is intense, but also brief. As cocaine levels in the brain drop, euphoria fades quickly and the user feels depressed and anxious with an intense desire to re-experience euphoria. The crack user becomes addicted quickly and soon realizes it is virtually impossible to overcome cravings for euphoria.

Crack cocaine first appeared in economically deprived areas of cities of the U.S. in 1985. This drug is known as "crack" on the East Coast and "rock" on the West Coast. Crack refers either to the crackling sound that crack makes when it is smoked or to pieces of plaster in tenement walls. This drug made a devastating impact from the start. Virtually the entire increase in murders in New York between 1985 and 1987 can be attributed to drug-related killings, specifically homicides associated with crack. Gangs throughout the city fought each other for control of the hot crack trade. In the three-year period from 1985 to 1987, the number of murders committed were, respectively, 1,384, 1,582, and 1,672 (Jonnes 1996; Lardner and Reppetto 2000; Saferstein 2001; Taylor 1988).

Other relatively new health hazards on the scene are designer drugs, designated as illegal substances in 1986. These include ecstasy, ketamine (also called special K), and GHB, among others. Designer drugs are illegally manufactured versions of already legally produced drugs. The chemical structure of these designer drugs tends to be slightly different from the legal equivalent, an alteration meant to protect the illegal manufacturer from prosecution under the Controlled Substance Act. Many designer drugs, including designer narcotics, are twenty to 2,000 times more potent than morphine, a powerful narcotic used to kill pain. Designer drugs can be toxic and can cause brain damage and death. Many of these drugs contain impurities that can induce seizures or psychoses. Users risk addiction and severe withdrawal (Aschenbrenner and Venable 2006; Drugs 1993; Lynton and Albertson 2004).

Most designer drug poisonings happen at raves or similar social events after these drugs have revved up the users. They dance for hours, perspiring and losing electrolytes—the chemicals and minerals required for a variety of essential body functions.

A popular rave drug, ecstasy is also known on the street as E, X, clarity, roll, and hug drug. Although a somewhat new addition to the recreational drug scene, this drug was first synthesized back in 1912 and patented in 1914 by the Merck Company in Germany as an appetite suppressant. In the 1960s, Alexander Shulgin, a biochemist with a Ph.D. from Berkeley, advocated the use of ecstasy as a psychotherapeutic agent. Since the 1980s, this drug has been increasingly abused; in 1985 it was classified in the U.S. as a Schedule I drug.

Available in 50-milligram to 150-milligram dosages, ecstasy tablets appear in different colors and are usually marked with an icon, typically the Motorola logo. These pills often contain adulterants such as aspirin and caffeine. This drug produces mild euphoria, increases energy, increases sexual desire, distorts the sense of time, and decreases thirst. Some users apply ecstasy to the inside of a surgical mask and inhale the drug. After a person takes ecstasy, about half an hour will pass before its effects are noticed. Subsequently, the effects rapidly increase and may last as long as eight hours. Snorting ecstasy powder produces a more rapid onset of effects.

Some people who ingest ecstasy orally develop a facial rash with reddish pimples. The distribution of pimples resembles periorificial dermatosis, an inflammatory skin disorder around the mouth, or an acne-like rash without whiteheads or blackheads. A side effect may be bruxism, the clenching or grinding of teeth. Some users rely on pacifiers to prevent any tooth damage.

Ecstasy is primarily metabolized in the liver. Overdose symptoms include a rapid heart rate (tachycardia), high blood pressure (hypertension), overheating of the body (hyperthermia), heavy perspiration (diaphoresis), and prolonged and abnormal dilation of the pupil (mydriasis).

In more severe cases, the user may die after a blood vessel ruptures in the head (intracerebral hemorrhage) and causes bleeding in the brain. Prior to death, this person may also experience heavy perspiration (diaphoresis) and abnormal heart rate (arrhythmia) (Buchanan and Brown 1988; Libiseller, Pavlic, Grubwieser, and Rabl 2005; Wollina, Kammler, Hesselbarth, Mock, and Bosseckert 1998).

The designer drug GHB was created for medicinal use, but is now abused by people seeking a high, as well as by rapists intent on incapacitating their victims. GHB is a naturally occurring acid produced by the human body and distributed in the central nervous system. Some scientists consider it to be a neurotransmitter, a chemical that transmits signals between nerve cells and the brain. GHB has a salty taste and is available as a white crystalline drug in capsules and tablets, as well as a colorless, odorless liquid manufactured by pharmaceutical companies.

Under the trade name Xyrem, GHB treats several medical conditions, including narcolepsy, a neurological disorder characterized by sudden, frequent, and uncontrollable episodes of sleep. GHB improves the length and quality of nocturnal REM (Rapid Eye Movement) sleep, the dreaming stage when the eyes move rapidly under the eyelids.

People at raves, all-night dance parties, or nightclubs have used illegally manufactured GHB since around 1994. Street names for GHB include Liquid X, Scoop, Liquid Ecstasy, and Cherry Meth. People who take GHB feel at ease socially and sexually. A person under the influence of GHB rapidly excretes it as carbon dioxide through exhalation. This is why GHB is not detected by routine urine or serum toxicology screens and is virtually undetectable in the urine twelve hours after ingestion.

One danger in taking this illegal drug is the lasting anterograde amnesia—the inability to transfer new events to long-term memory—regarding events that took place while the user was under the influence. This is why GHB is a date-rape drug. Another danger in taking the illegal drug is the uncertainty of dosage.

Users buy this drug in bars, over the Internet, and in gyms, where it is used as an alternative to steroids for muscle building and weight control. In the 1980s, GHB was sold to consumers in the U.S. as a dietary supplement. After taking into account reports of abuse and adverse effects, in 1990 the Food and Drug Administration declared all products containing GHB to be unsafe. Sale of these products to the public was banned.

Users may develop a tolerance for GHB and become addicted. Chronic heavy users can experience severe withdrawal, resembling withdrawal from alcohol, and may have psychotic symptoms, including visual hallucinations. Overdosing on GHB causes nausea, vomiting, disorientation, convulsions, and coma. An especially deadly activity is to drink alcoholic beverages while using GHB. This may depress respiration to the degree that the user dies.

In 1999, the death of a young teen brought the hazards of this drug to national attention. Three young men in Detroit, Michigan, were convicted of involuntary manslaughter after a fifteen-year-old girl was given GHB in a soft drink without her knowledge and died next day. Her death inspired the

Hillory J. Farias and Samantha Reid Date-Rape Prohibition Act of 2000, legislating GHB as a Schedule I Controlled Substance. A Schedule I substance does not have accepted medical use in the U.S. and has a high abuse potential (Bernstein 2004; Jones 2001; Nicholson and Balster 2001; Schwartz, Milteer, and LeBeau 2000; Tarabar and Nelson 2004).

Developed in 1963, ketamine is a tasteless, odorless, and colorless drug used in human anesthesia and veterinary medicine. It maintains respiration and blood pressure in human patients in critical care. Veterinarians use ketamine to sedate animals for travel, surgery, and euthanasia. Legally prescribed, this drug is a liquid that can be ingested or injected. Illegal ketamine used in clubs is taken intra-nasally with a nasal inhaler or as a powder smoked in a mixture of marijuana or tobacco. Keets, jet, Special K, vitamin K, and kit-kat are a few of ketamine's street names.

A dissociative anesthetic, ketamine distorts the user's perceptions of sight and sound and produces feelings of detachment from the environment and from the user's own self. Ketamine was derived from phencyclidine (PCP), a drug used as an anesthetic by veterinarians. Medical use of ketamine is limited because its side effects include bizarre ideations and hallucinations, which appeal to recreational drug users.

The recreational ketamine user experiences a feeling of floating outside the body, visual hallucinations, and a dreamlike state within thirty to forty-five minutes of ingestion. Like the GHB user, this user may also experience anterograde amnesia as well as hypertension, apnea, and palpitations. Flashbacks, vivid memories in which the user feels like she is re-experiencing a former ketamine high, may appear days or weeks later; people who continue to abuse ketamine may become severely addicted. Sexual predators reportedly have used this drug to incapacitate their victims, either by lacing drinks with the drug or by giving it to victims without letting them know the drug's full effects (Gahlinger 2004).

Another popular recreational and potential date-rape drug, Rohypnol (flunitrazepam), is also known by the street names roofies, circles, rope, and forget-me pill. Medically, it's a psychotropic drug used as an antianxiety agent, muscle relaxant, sedative, and treatment for insomnia. Rohypnol is approximately ten times as potent as Valium and can be injected or taken as 1-milligram and 2-milligram tablets. Rohypnol's half-life, or the time it takes for half of the dose to be metabolized in the body, is approximately twenty hours.

High doses of this drug can cause lack of muscle control and loss of consciousness. Alcohol and other sedating drugs increase Rohypnol's potency; people who consume this combination may experience amnesia and lose their inhibitions. One milligram can impair a person for eight to twelve hours, with sedation occurring within thirty minutes of ingestion. Adverse effects include low blood pressure (hypotension), confusion, visual disturbances, and urinary retention. Detection methods commonly fail because

Rohypnol is administered in small amounts and is rapidly distributed in the body. GCMS (gas chromatography-mass spectrometry) can detect a 1-milligram dose up to seventy-two hours after ingestion (Gahlinger 2004).

Some people inhale vapors or gases that produce psychoactive (mind-altering) and aphrodisiac effects. Their drug of choice may in fact be the emissions from common household products such as paint thinner, hair spray, model airplane glue, or gasoline. One common inhalant with medical use is nitrous oxide, or "laughing gas," a colorless and odorless gas used as an anesthetic and analgesic. High concentrations produce a narcotic effect and may cause death by asphyxia—a lack of oxygen followed by suffocation.

The usual techniques for consuming inhalants are sniffing; drawing in the vapors through the mouth ("huffing"); spraying the inhalant into a plastic or paper bag and then pulling the bag over one's head and huffing; painting nails with correction fluid and inhaling the fumes; or spraying an aerosol substance into the mouth. Inhalants temporarily stimulate the central nervous system and cause confusion, dizziness, reduced coordination, tachycardia (abnormally rapid heartbeat), and hallucinations. The high from inhalants is brief, usually lasting about half an hour.

Signs of inhalant abuse include redness around the mouth and nose, red or runny eyes or nose, and breath with a chemical odor. Long-term use can lead to weight loss, fatigue, and muscle weakness. Inhaling toxic substances may lead to sudden heart failure or respiratory failure followed by death. A user may have sudden heart failure if he is caught in the act of inhaling or if she experiences a frightening hallucination. A person using inhalants can also die from a fire-related injury if a cigarette is lit in a closed area filled with inhalant vapors and the inhalant combusts.

In 2002, approximately 180,000 Americans were dependent on or abused inhalants. Children and teenagers who are anxious, depressed, and angry abuse inhalants, as do adults as old as fifty or sixty. This includes nurses, dentists, hairstylists, and dry-cleaning workers—all of whom are at risk for inhalant abuse due to the availability of these products in their workplaces (Aschenbrenner and Venable 2006; Drugs 1993; Guidelines 2006).

More illegal drugs than can be covered here are currently on the market. As many people are willing to take these unregulated products made by anonymous, illegal manufacturers, medical examiners must be aware of what the results of these substances look like on the autopsy table.

6

---·•·---

DEATH BY VENOM AND POISON

BECAUSE OF THE great variety of toxic substances in the world, investigating poisoning deaths can be a challenge, particularly when the poison is obscure. If the medical examiner finds no clue to point him or the toxicologist in the right direction, the killing poison could be missed. In this chapter, we'll cover a few of the more common types of poisonings, as well as the types of venom an ME may encounter in his work.

Radiation poisoning is a rare type of poisoning that could threaten a medical examiner's health during a death investigation. Many medical examiners, if not most, would prefer not to perform an autopsy on a person who died of radiation poisoning, as the body could continue to be radioactive and could hurt the ME. For this reason, some people are buried without undergoing an autopsy, even though an autopsy could reveal important medical information.

A recent news-making example of death by radiation poisoning happened in November 2006 in England. Alexander Litvinenko, a forty-three-year-old former KGB agent and vocal critic of Russian President Vladimir Putin, died after being poisoned by polonium-210, a radioactive element. Polonium, discovered in 1898 by Marie Curie and her husband, Pierre, is more than 400 times as radioactive as uranium (Spy 2006).

Before he died, Litvinenko left a radiation trail connected to twelve contaminated sites, including two hospitals and a hotel; his autopsy required the forensic pathologist to wear radiation protection, according to an article published December 1, 2006, in *USA Today*, "Radioactive Traces Found at 12 Sites in Spy Probe; Autopsy Friday."

When investigating a suspected poisoning death, the medical examiner notes any unusual odors emanating from the dead person's mouth, as well as changes in the color and texture of the person's skin. For example, skin that is gray and scaly, with a rash on the palms of the hands and on the soles of the feet, points to thallium poisoning. Thallium is used to kill rats and ants. A faint odor of bitter almonds indicates death by potassium cyanide poisoning. This poison looks like table salt; a killer may mix it with other white substances before serving it to a victim (Kaye 1995). A garlic-like odor may indicate arsenic in the body, while a blue-black gumline may indicate mercury or lead poisoning.

Some poisons seem to be everywhere. Cyanide is an extremely toxic poison found in numerous processes and substances, including metal treatment operations, thermal decomposition of polyurethane foam, tobacco smoke, and certain drugs such as laetrile. Laetrile is prepared from the pits of apricots or peaches and, although purportedly a cure for cancer, is banned by the Food and Drug Administration. Cyanide is a quick-acting poison and must be handled cautiously, as it can enter the body orally or through skin contact, mucous membranes, and inhalation. Cyanide produces tissue hypoxia (reduction of oxygen supply) or anoxia (absence of oxygen supply). It disturbs the central nervous system and heart, and binds irreversibly to hemoglobin, the oxygen-carrying component of red blood cells. This leaves hemoglobin unable to transport oxygen.

A victim of cyanide poisoning becomes dizzy, confused, and nauseous;\ staggers; and loses consciousness. At autopsy, the victim will have pinkish spots on the skin, an indication of oxygen deprivation. The medical examiner also notes these types of spots in victims of carbon monoxide poisoning. The ME may smell a bitter almond odor emanating from the victim's mouth. Cyanide in a body breaks down into carbon and nitrogen; no trace of cyanide remains after a few days (*MacMillan* 1997; Ramsland 2005).

Some people become medical examiner cases after they use sabotaged over-the-counter drugs. In one case of product tampering, a medical examiner discovered lethal levels of cyanide in forty-year-old Kathleen Daneker's body fluids after the Tacoma, Washington, resident died on February 11, 1991. Just a week later, a medical examiner found more deadly amounts of cyanide in forty-four-year-old Stanley McWhorter, a Lacey, Washington, resident who died February 18. The medical examiner's office learned of a telling coincidence: Daneker and McWhorter had both taken Sudafed 12-hour cold relief capsules purchased near their homes.

Police and medical examiners linked these deaths to a 911 call on February 2 from Joseph Meling, thirty-one, of Tumwater, Washington. Meling, a former sales agent with the Prudential Insurance Company in Lacey, had told the 911 operator that his wife, Jennifer Meling, became unconscious after ingesting a Sudafed capsule at their apartment. Meling suggested to doctors that they check her for cyanide poisoning. Doctors indeed found cyanide in her blood—although she did not die. FBI agents in the investigation discovered that on January 11 that year, Meling bought a pound of sodium cyanide for eleven dollars at the Emerald City Chemical Company in Kent, Washington. He used a false Washington state driver's license as identification to make the purchase (Washington State's Toxic Substance Registry requires anyone buying a toxic chemical to show identification to a sales clerk).

It wasn't long before the FBI uncovered Meling's plot—and the irony that had him convicted for causing two deaths while his true target survived. Although a blue band sealing Sudafed capsule shells makes them tamper-resistant, the generic capsules Meling used did not have this seal and came apart easily. Meling tucked his cyanide-laced capsules in blister packs, placed them in Sudafed packages, and returned the cyanide-laced medicine to store shelves.

His intention: to deflect attention from himself while he murdered his spouse and collected $700,000 in life insurance money. Meling knew other cyanide-laced capsules would be found and the police would have Sudafed recalled. If his wife had died, her death would have been attributed to tampering. Meling was indicted on April 21, 1992, and was sentenced in 1993 to two concurrent life terms and seventy-five years in prison for product tampering and for causing the deaths of Daneker and McWhorter (Ropp 1993).

Some types of poisonings tend to be more accidental than others, such as carbon monoxide poisoning. Every year people seek refuge from the cold in a motor vehicle while keeping the engine running, sometimes while it's parked in a building or perhaps waiting in deep snow. This can create lethal levels of carbon monoxide (CO) in the vehicle or building, accidentally killing the occupants. Of course, some people commit suicide or murder this way.

Carbon monoxide is an odorless, tasteless, colorless, and nonirritating gas. It has been known as a toxic substance since the third century B.C. Sources of carbon monoxide include incompletely combusted coal, oil, and natural gas. Other sources of CO are automobile, truck, and airplane exhaust gases, as well as emissions from furnaces and space heaters.

When a person inhales carbon monoxide, it bonds with hemoglobin 200 to 240 times more effectively than does oxygen. This reduces the oxygen-carrying capacity of blood, so tissues receive less oxygen than required for the body to properly function. The more carbon monoxide replaces oxygen in cells, the greater the disruption of cellular metabolism and the eventual death of cells. The CO concentration level matters: a person in an environment where carbon monoxide concentrations are 35 parts per million (ppm) will not suffer adverse effects within eight hours. A person will lose consciousness after one hour when concentrations are 1,000 ppm. Unconsciousness and the danger of death follow after a person is exposed to concentrations of 12,800 ppm for only one to three minutes.

Physical symptoms of CO poisoning are headache, dizziness, and nausea; psychological symptoms include difficulty thinking and hallucinations. The nose or nails of a number of people who have carbon monoxide poisoning will turn cherry red or bright pink.

Carbon monoxide poisoning can be a silent killer. U.S. tennis player Vitas Gerulaitis died on September 18, 1994, in Long Island, New York, while he slept in a friend's cottage. The forty-year-old athlete died from exposure to

CO fumes from an improperly installed heater. In 1996, a Suffolk County jury acquitted Bartholomew Torpey, a thirty-four-year-old pool mechanic, of criminally negligent homicide (Carbon Monoxide 2004; Fallon 2004; Ilano and Raffin 2004; Kales 2004; Mechanic 2004; Safety 2004).

Pesticides are another type of poison that can lurk in the environment. These toxins are perhaps the most ordinary kind of poison: they're used in gardens, in homes and offices, and in agriculture. But chemicals used to kill pests can also kill people, and pesticides may adversely affect human health through residues on food crops.

The Environmental Protection Agency monitors pesticide residues in domestically produced food. The Food and Drug Administration and the U.S. Department of Agriculture also sample approximately 1 percent of the national food supply for pesticide residues. Meanwhile, the Federal Insecticide, Fungicide, and Rodenticide Act (FIRA) of 1947, amended numerous times since then, helps determine if a pesticide should be discontinued. In 2004, the U.S. accounted for more than 25 percent of the worldwide pesticide market. This global market sees more than 1,600 pesticides, about 4.4 million tons used annually worldwide, at an annual cost of more than $20 billion.

Yet with all the bug-killing toxins being used today, fewer people are dying as a direct result of pesticide poisonings. In 1969, pesticides could not be excluded as the cause in eighty-seven deaths. Sixty-two of these deaths were accidental; twenty deaths were intentional; five deaths were incorrectly attributed to pesticides. The eighty-seven deaths indicated a downward trend compared to deaths during the period spanning 1947–1962. An important finding in three of the deaths in 1969 revealed that intensive inhalation of aerosol cans caused fatal arrhythmia in the hearts of people who did not intentionally misuse the aerosol. Pesticide mortality continued to decrease during 1979–1998.

Rates of suicide by pesticide dropped more slowly in this time period, but these suicides did not necessarily occur where pesticides are regularly used. Pesticides may pose another kind of health threat—statistics show that agricultural workers are at greater risk of accidental mortality from cancers of the blood and nervous system.

Research reported in 1983 showed four deaths from methyl bromide, an insecticide fumigant, in Dade County, Florida. Afflicted individuals experienced a variety of symptoms, including nausea, vomiting, malaise, seizures, and delirium prior to respiratory failure. At autopsy, the medical examiner saw abnormal buildup of fluid in the lungs (pulmonary edema), inflammation of the air sacs in the lungs (alveolitis), and accumulation of excessive fluid in the brain (cerebral edema) (Fleming, Gomez-Marin, Zheng, Ma, and Lee 2003; Hayes 1976; Langley and Sumner 2002; Maddy, Edmiston, and Richmond 1990; Marraccini, Thomas, Ongley, Pfaffenberger, Davis, and Bednarczyk 1983).

On the topic of gardening, some common garden plants have highly toxic elements, in particular the castor bean. The plant's humble brown, mottled, oblong beans are used to make castor oil, a product found in varnishes, paint, and lubricant for jet engines and industrial machinery. Castor oil can also be used as a purgative; it's not thought to contain poison. But the bean pulp left over after the oil is removed contains ricin, a highly toxic substance. The act of chewing these beans will generally release the poison. Some reports suggest eight beans is the lethal dose, although death is associated with as few as two beans (Audi, Belson, Patel, Schier, and Osterloh 2005).

Purified ricin is a water-soluble white powder; poisoning can occur through ingestion, inhalation, or injection—and possibly on the point of an umbrella. Evidence suggests this toxin was used in the 1978 assassination of Bulgarian broadcaster Georgi Markov in England. Markov survived long enough to tell his wife that while waiting for the bus, he felt a sharp jab into the back of his right thigh. Turning, he saw a man drop an umbrella. Once home, Markov became ill and was soon hospitalized. He died on the third day following the incident. In the autopsy, a tiny metallic sphere the size of a pinhead was removed from under the broadcaster's skin at the umbrella-point wound site. This sphere had two minuscule holes crossing in the center—presumably to hold the toxin. Dr. David Gall at the Government Chemical Defense Establishment at Porton Down studied the sphere and, although he could not isolate the poison, he was satisfied that it was likely ricin. He reached this determination both because of the symptoms and because of the toxic potency of such a small dose (Knight 1979).

Someone who has ingested ricin may suffer a variety of symptoms within twelve hours, including nausea, vomiting, diarrhea, and abdominal pain. In severe cases the person may develop hypotension (low blood pressure), liver failure, renal dysfunction, and eventually may die from multi-organ failure or cardiovascular collapse. A person who inhales aerosol formulations with ricin may expect to see symptoms within eight hours, including cough, dyspnea, arthralgias, and fever; a person with a severe case may suffer respiratory distress and die.

Ricin was discovered in White House mail in 2001, a South Carolina postal facility in 2003, and U.S. Senator Bill Frist's office in 2004. Researchers are studying ricin as a potential biological threat, while the Centers for Disease Control and Prevention have categorized the poison as a Category B agent, the second highest priority. No vaccine or antidote currently exists to prevent or treat ricin poisoning. Prompt medical treatment is essential to save lives; the key is for health care workers and public health officials to consider ricin poisoning as a possibility when people develop gastrointestinal or respiratory tract illnesses in public settings. In autopsy, the medical examiner will likely find diffuse intestinal hemorrhagic lesions in a person who died from ricin poisoning (Audi, Belson, Patel, Schier, and Osterloh 2005).

Household products can be highly toxic if misused, either unintentionally or otherwise. Three U.S. Air Force airmen used Liquid Drano as an assault weapon in 1974 in Ogden, Utah. On April 22, the airmen forced two women and three men in the Hi-Fi Shop to drink Liquid Drano. Ingestion of the Drano produced blisters, burned tongue, and throats, and destroyed skin around the victims' mouths. Pierre Selby, one of the airmen, then shot the victims in the head. Carol Naisbitt, Stanley Walker, and Michelle Ansley died. Cortney Naisbitt and Orren Walker survived. Airmen Selby and William Andrews were put to death by lethal injection in 1987 and 1992, respectively. The third airman, Keith Roberts, was imprisoned until 1987 (Hi-Fi Murders 2006).

Animals carry their own types of poisons, called "venom." Snakes, scorpions, ants, bees, and spiders are among the long list of creatures with some kind of toxic weapon. The U.S. alone is home to approximately twenty indigenous venomous snakes, almost all of which are pit vipers: venomous snakes with heat-sensitive pits below their eyes that are used to detect prey. Cottonmouths, copperheads, and rattlesnakes are pit vipers. The coral snake is the only venomous snake indigenous to the U.S. that is not a pit viper.

While there are between 7,000 and 8,000 venomous snakebites annually in the U.S., only five or six bites per year lead to death. Typical victims of venomous snakebites are intoxicated males aged seventeen to twenty-seven. Most are bitten on the hands or arms when they attempt to handle, harm, or kill a snake. Other common victims include children and the elderly.

Twenty-five percent of pit viper bites are "dry," meaning no venom is injected into a victim. The most fatalities are caused by the eastern and western diamondback rattlesnakes. The eastern diamondback is the largest rattlesnake in the U.S. and may grow up to eight feet in length. It lives in underground cavities, including gopher burrows. These snakes live on the coastal plain from North Carolina to Mississippi and in all of Florida. Eastern diamondbacks feed on rabbits, squirrels, and birds (Gold, Dart, and Barish 2002).

The western diamondback may grow more than seven feet in length. Like the eastern diamondback, it also lives in underground cavities. The western diamondback is found in diverse habitats, including desert flats and grassy plains in parts of Arkansas, Texas, Oklahoma, Arizona, and California. Its diet includes rats and chipmunks.

Puncture wounds and scratches characterize pit viper bites. Within half an hour to an hour, the victim experiences, at the bite site and in surrounding tissue, pain, edema, erythema (redness of the skin caused by dilation and congestion of the capillaries), or ecchymosis (passage of blood from ruptured blood vessels into subcutaneous tissue with purple discoloration of the skin).

Other indicators of a pit viper bite include nausea, vomiting, tingling of the fingertips and toes, continuous involuntary muscle twitching, lethargy, low blood pressure, rapid breathing, and an abnormally rapid heartbeat (over 100 beats per minute) while the victim is at rest. The venom destroys living tissue and red blood cells; kidney failure may result from low blood pressure; and the victim may have hypovolemic shock: shock caused by severe blood and fluid loss that prevents the heart from pumping the required amount of blood through the body. Pit viper bites are almost immediately fatal if venom directly enters a vein.

Rattlesnakes are also potentially dangerous—but, again, few people die from rattlesnake bites. During the period of 1900 to 1991 in Utah, only five people died from rattlesnake bites, according to death certificates at the Utah Bureau of Health Statistics (Straight and Glenn 1993).

A better understanding of death from rattlesnake venom in the U.S. comes from data about Arizona. A review of death certificates for Arizona for the years 1969–1984 indicated that nine people—six males and three females aged two to seventy-seven years—died of fatal rattlesnake bites. Prolonged hypotension (abnormally low blood pressure) and organ failure apparently caused the deaths. Causes of death included cardiac failure; renal failure; unconsciousness with airway obstruction and brain damage; and coagulopathy (blood clotting disorder) with multiple hemorrhage sites.

Most of the nine deaths might have been prevented had the victims not delayed going to a medical facility where antivenin either was not administered promptly or was administered in inadequate amounts. The victims also needed to have their low blood pressure treated (Hardy 1986).

One highly unusual method of suicide is to deliberately inject oneself with snake venom. This method was reported by Bernard Knight of the Welsh National School of Medicine in Cardiff, Wales, and Andrew Barclay and Roger Mann of the Home Office Forensic Science Laboratory in Birmingham, England. They studied the death of a twenty-six-year-old male schizophrenic who committed suicide by injecting himself with a syringe containing snake venom.

The victim had talked for years about committing suicide. He overdosed on drugs at age fifteen and again at twenty-three. In the latter attempt, he took nitrazepam, also known by the trade name Mogadon. This drug is used to control seizures and treat insomnia. While in a psychiatric hospital, the victim's blood pressure increased, his pulse became rapid, and he claimed he was very thirsty. He admitted to a doctor that he had injected himself with snake venom. He was transferred to a general hospital and treated with an anti-serum to European snakes before he lapsed into a coma and died the next morning.

During the external examination at the autopsy, an injection mark and petechial hemorrhages were noted on the man's left forearm. During the internal examination, all the blood, although extremely dark and somewhat hemolyzed (broken down), was noted to be completely fluid. The lungs were very congested. The stomach and intestines contained dark red bloodstained fluid. The vessels of the renal medulla, the innermost part of the kidney, were extensively congested and appeared almost black. Laboratory investigation indicated the victim had possibly injected himself with a mixture of two venoms, or venom with two properties that cause death. Part of the venom present in the man's tissue was North American rattlesnake venom (Knight, Barclay, and Mann 1977).

In the U.S., as reported in the *Southern Medical Journal* in 2006, a fourteen-year-old male attempted to commit suicide by injecting himself with rattlesnake venom in a vein in his right arm. He experienced pain immediately and vomited. He developed hypotension and swollen lips and tongue, followed by coma. Over twenty-four hours he had gastrointestinal bleeding and blood in his urine (hematuria). After receiving antivenin and spending five days in the hospital, he was discharged (Morgan, Blair, and Ramsey 2006).

Snake venom has also been used to commit murder, although in the following case, the official attending the scene failed to recognize the snakebite—or the homicide.

In June 1935 in Los Angeles, California, Robert James, a barber known to use money from life insurance policies for sexual escapades, was cutting Charles Hope's hair on credit. James, forty, told Hope that a friend needed two rattlesnakes to fatally bite his wife. The barber promised to give Hope one hundred dollars if Hope would provide the rattlesnakes. The friend wanting to kill his wife was James himself.

Hope bought two vipers from a herpetologist, Snake Joe Houtenbrink. James tested the vipers by putting them into a cage with chickens; the snakes bit the chickens, and the chickens died. Satisfied that the rattlesnakes would kill his wife, James gave Hope one hundred dollars.

On August 4, James persuaded Mary James, his most recent wife, to have an abortion on the kitchen table of their home. She drank several ounces of whiskey as an "anesthetic." She allowed her eyes and mouth to be taped shut because abortion was illegal and the "doctor," Hope, did not want to be recognized. Hope entered the kitchen carrying a box that had a sliding glass door. He opened the door, James put Mary's left leg into the box, and a snake bit the leg. Hope left with the two snakes and sold them for half price to Houtenbrink.

Mary James's leg swelled to twice its normal size and turned purple. By evening she was still alive, writhing in pain on the kitchen table as James and Hope sat in the garage drinking whiskey. Impatient that she was taking too long to die, James carried his wife into the bathroom and drowned her in the bathtub, as he had drowned a previous wife.

At about 6 A.M. the next day, James and Hope carried Mary James outside and placed her body headfirst into the fishpond, staging the crime scene to look as if she had tripped, fallen in, and drowned. The coroner who attended the scene decided an insect bite had caused Mary James's death.

That same month the owner of a liquor store told a Los Angeles *Herald-Express* reporter that a man he knew, whose last name was Hope, told him about buying and testing rattlesnakes and then using them to bite a pregnant woman. He added that the man said the woman was drowned in a bathtub and then left in a fishpond outside because the snake venom did not kill her.

The reporter told Chief Deputy District Attorney Eugene Williams about Hope. Police and insurance investigators uncovered some of James's past misdeeds, and Hope testified against James. One of James's lovers testified he offered her money to be his alibi on the day Mary James died. Eventually, both men were convicted of first-degree murder. Hope received a life sentence; James received the death penalty. On May 1, 1942, Robert James was the last person in California to be executed by hanging (Wolf and Mader 1986).

Swimmers, snorkelers, and scuba divers may encounter venomous fish such as stingrays. A stingray has winglike fins and a horizontally flattened body with gills on its underside. It also has a barbed spine near the base of a whiplike tail that can inflict severe wounds. A stingray that feels threatened will use its tail to strike the victim, penetrating or lacerating the victim's skin. Its stinger, the razor-sharp spine coated with venom, grows from its tail up to thirty-seven centimeters in length.

Stingray venom contains toxic proteins that include serotonin, a neurotransmitter (chemical messenger) that constricts blood vessels at injury sites and may affect human emotions. Because serotonin produces severe and immediate local pain, a sting that is free from pain indicates that poison did not enter the wound. Stingray venom may produce local and/or systemic effects, including vomiting, sweating, convulsions, abdominal pain, and cardiac arrhythmia (irregular heartbeat).

In the U.S., more than 1,500 people are stung annually, mostly on their legs, but deaths from stings are rare (How 2006). However, on September 4, 2006, Steve Irwin, the Australian known worldwide for his television series, *Crocodile Hunter*, was killed off the coast of Australia by a stingray's sting to his heart while filming a documentary.

Scorpions are similar to stingrays in that they have stingers on their tails. But the venom of one American species of scorpion is perhaps better compared to that of a rattlesnake. Found in Arizona and surrounding states, the bark scorpion is a fraction of the size of a rattlesnake, yet its venom is just as deadly. A small tooth at the base of the bark scorpion's stinger distinguishes this scorpion from others. Generally nocturnal, this creature hides under rocks and leaves and hibernates during the winter. The bark scorpion stings when handled or otherwise threatened. A person who is stung will experience paresthesia—a burning, tickling, or prickling sensation, usually in the hands, arms, legs, or feet. A severe sting can cause difficulty in breathing, irregular heartbeat, and death.

Nevertheless, deaths from scorpion stings are rare, and the stings of other species of scorpions don't usually cause systemic reactions. Records show 1968 was the last year a death from a bark scorpion was reported in the U.S. (Covington 2003).

In the southeastern U.S., the most common cause of allergy due to insect venom is from stings by a red imported fire ant. The body's first reaction to a sting is a flare, an area of redness, of up to two inches wide that appears immediately around the sting. Next a wheal, a raised area of skin, rises. This is almost always an indicator of allergy. Within ninety minutes, small bumps show, followed by pustules—collections of pus in the top layer of skin—within twenty-four hours. Pustules remain for a few days to more than a week. They eventually rupture and leave a crust, and sometimes a scar. In severe cases, skin grafts or limb amputations may be necessary. An injured or intoxicated person who falls on a mound of red imported fire ants may become the insects' next meal.

Another way people can be seriously harmed or die from fire ant stings is through a severe allergic reaction known as *anaphylactic shock*. Symptoms include fever, dizziness, vomiting, unconsciousness, reduced heart rate, and a swollen larynx. Anaphylactic shock requires immediate emergency treatment. In 1985, about forty million people in the U.S. lived within contact of these ants. Rates of death are low compared to the number who are stung, but are significant—fourteen million people are stung annually, and about one hundred of them die every year.

From a medical examiner's perspective, a fire ant sting is the cause of death when a witness has direct knowledge of an attack; the decedent had a history of hypersensitivity to fire ant stings; evidence of anaphylaxis exists; the body has enzyme elevated blood tryptase; the body has elevated venom-specific antibody levels; and nothing else can explain the decedent's death. Some medical examiners report a death by anaphylaxis, such as after a red imported fire ant sting, as a natural death because of deficiencies in the decedent's immune system. Other medical examiners deem this type of death accidental, as these ants are part of the environment and chance is a factor in the encounter between ant and person (Taber 2000).

Bee stings can also result in anaphylactic shock. In the U.S., one species of bee is more likely to sting than all others: Africanized honey bees, also known as killer bees. An unusually aggressive species, this bee may attack when unprovoked and will do so in large numbers. Severe allergic reactions have occurred in some people after one or more stings. These bees are recent arrivals from South America. In October 1990, the first Africanized honey bees arrived in the Lower Rio Grande Valley; they've been in California since 1995.

Deaths caused by massive poisoning and toxic effects—without allergic reactions—have also been reported from these bee stings. Toxicity from thirty to fifty stings has killed children. In severely stung victims, the stings' high toxicity causes the breakdown of red blood cells (cells that transport oxygen) and the breakdown of muscle fibers, leading to the toxic release of muscle contents into the blood.

A person who has been stung multiple times can experience immediate as well as delayed toxic reactions. Nausea, vomiting, and kidney failure are signs of an immediate toxic reaction. A person may also initially experience only pain, but then eighteen hours later exhibit signs of organ failure. This person's blood may be unable to form a clot (coagulopathy), and there may be an abnormal decrease in the number of platelets in circulating blood (thrombocytopenia). Death may follow without medical attention (Bresolin, Carvalho, Goes, Fernandes, and Barotto 2002; Kolecki 1999; McKenna 1992).

Spiders inspire fear in many individuals, but most arachnids are relatively harmless to people. An exception is the brown recluse spider, commonly found in the Southeast and the Central Midwest U.S. As its name implies, this spider is shy, and usually only bites when it is trapped in a person's clothing or when its nest is disturbed. Most bites have no symptoms, although in three or four days the location of a bite may show necrosis, a form of cell death in which cells become swollen, break apart, and release their contents into neighboring tissues. This may damage cells and cause inflammation. Ulcers at this location may be difficult to heal and may require skin grafting or amputation of the bitten area. Rare victims may die after experiencing nausea, fever, rashes, and the breakdown of blood cells (Forks 2000; Merigian and Blaho 1996; Nunnelee 2006).

Although mosquito bites are not venomous, a mosquito can transmit a virus that can kill a person. Mosquitoes, mostly *Culex* mosquitoes, will feed off birds, particularly crows, ravens, and jays, that may be infected with West Nile virus (WNV). This dangerous virus incubates for approximately three to fourteen days before the mosquitoes can transfer it to people. Although it can't be received through person-to-person transmission, a person can also be infected with the virus through a blood transfusion or organ transplant from infected donors, as well as through breastfeeding. The virus invades living cells to survive and reproduces itself during summer and fall in North America.

WNV was discovered in birds in New York City in 1999 and was linked by the Centers for Disease Control (CDC) with a human encephalitis outbreak that year. Prior to the 1999 outbreak, WNV had not been seen in birds or people in the Western Hemisphere. WNV was named for the area in Uganda where it was discovered in 1937.

West Nile virus can cause several life-threatening diseases: West Nile encephalitis, an inflammation of the brain; West Nile meningitis, an inflammation of the membrane around the brain and spinal cord; and West Nile meningoencephalitis, an inflammation of the brain and its surrounding membranes. Laboratory confirmation for antibodies to the virus in serum or cerebrospinal fluid will confirm the virus is present in a person's body. About 20 percent of people bitten by an infected mosquito will have mild symptoms such as fever, headache, vomiting, and a skin rash on the chest or back. These symptoms usually last a few days, and medical attention is not required. Individuals over age fifty with weak immune systems are at the greatest risk of dying. Indicators of a severe case of WNV disease are high fever, headache, vision loss, convulsions, and slurred, slow, and garbled speech (dysarthria).

During an autopsy of a severe case of WNV, a forensic pathologist may find a viral infection of the spinal cord that caused flaccid paralysis; heart muscle inflammation (myocarditis); kidney inflammation (nephritis); and the presence of West Nile virus in the decedent's mid-brain tissue. In 2002, the CDC received 4,156 reports of human disease cases due to WNV in forty-four states. Approximately 3,000 were central nervous system (CNS) cases; others suffered from West Nile fever. Of the cases involving the CNS, about 300 were fatal (Jeha and Sila 2004; Petersen and Marfin 2002).

Of course, there are too many varieties of venom and poison to cover in this chapter—in fact, an entire book on this topic may not be enough. But while the list of available lethal toxins is long, the medical examiner has some advantages in detecting a particular toxin over his colleagues who treat live patients. First, the patient is already dead, so some of the pressure is off when it comes to waiting for toxicology results. Second, a medical examiner can perform a thorough autopsy to physically search for hidden, underlying causes and contributors to the death.

In this case, the answers will be on and in the body.

7

DEATH BY SUICIDE

THE STATISTICS ON suicide may surprise you: every eighteen minutes, someone in the U.S. takes his or her own life. Thirty thousand Americans die this way every year. More than half of these victims are men between the ages of twenty-five and sixty-five; in fact, males are four times more likely to kill themselves than females (Henkel 2005).

After attending suicide scenes year after year, medical examiners often see the same details time and again. For example, women rarely commit suicide in the nude; men are more likely to use weapons; women are more likely to use poison; a suicidal drowning victim usually leaves her hat, coat, and wallet behind and then jumps feet first into the water; and a suicidal person rarely shoots himself in the eye. As an aside, a person shot in the eye is more likely to have been murdered by an underworld killer who uses a small caliber gun than by his own hand. Shooting through the eye ensures the bullet ricochets inside the skull and produces permanent brain damage (Schultz 1978).

Some suicides are so public, there can be no doubt the victims died by their own hands. For example, Christine Chubbuck, twenty-nine, was the host of a television talk show in Sarasota, Florida. On July 15, 1974, on live television, she put a .38 revolver to her head and pulled the trigger. Fourteen hours later, she was pronounced dead at Sarasota Memorial Hospital (Christine 2006).

In late 1986, forty-seven-year-old R. Budd Dwyer, the state treasurer of Pennsylvania, was charged with receiving a kickback of $300,000. The kickback was associated with a $4.6 million contract awarded to Computer Technology Associates and its owner, John Torquato, Jr. Dwyer, who professed his innocence and refused a plea bargain, faced sentencing of up to fifty-five years in prison and a fine of $300,000. On January 22, 1987, the day before his sentencing, and during a press conference on live television, he reached into an envelope, removed a .357 Magnum revolver, put it into his mouth, and pulled the trigger. He was pronounced dead at the scene

(Morris 1987; Pennsylvania Officials 1987; Pennsylvania Official Kills 1987).

In another type of public suicide, suicide-by-cop, the victims do nothing directly to kill themselves. Instead, the person wields a weapon, refuses to drop it when confronted by police, may threaten the life of police officers or others nearby, and is then shot dead, sometimes after taunting police to shoot. This type of person wants to die but is incapable of killing herself. One case is that of Deborah J. Meyer, a thirty-one-year-old from Milwaukee, Wisconsin. On January 28, 1999, Meyer entered a convenience store and began waving a handgun. Police arrived and ordered her to drop her weapon. Instead, she pointed the gun at one of the officers. Four officers fired fourteen rounds at her, and Meyer was pronounced dead about an hour later at St. Catherine's Hospital. Her suicide notes were found later (Cole 1999).

To a medical examiner, the above suicides are relatively clear-cut. The victims' names are known, their cause of death is clear, the manner of death is obvious, and there are numerous witnesses. The vast majority of suicides are not committed in public, however. Investigators at death scenes must determine with great care if the deaths were suicides or homicides.

Shooting oneself is the most common method of suicide, especially by men. Handguns are more likely to be used in urban communities, long guns in rural communities. A person who uses a handgun usually places it in one of six areas on the body before pulling the trigger: in the mouth, side of the forehead, front of the forehead, behind the ear, to the temple, or to the heart. A long gun is usually positioned to fire upward, the muzzle placed under the chin, at the forehead, or in the mouth, or is pointed downward into either the lower or upper area of the chest. In calling the death a suicide, the medical examiner must determine how the victim of a long gun shot was able to pull the trigger. If the victim could not have reached the trigger, the death was a disguised homicide.

Sometimes people who commit suicide with guns—particularly with smaller guns—will graze themselves before they fire the fatal shot. It's also possible for a person to shoot herself twice due to cadaveric spasm (a type of near-instant rigor mortis that grips the body or parts of the body, typically after exertion; see Chapter 2). She may initially appear to be a homicide victim, but a medical examiner will soon learn that the death was a suicide.

Self-inflicted fatal gunshot wounds almost always indicate suicide, even though the family of the victim may deny that the death was a suicide, and tell police and the medical examiner that a gun cleaning accident was the cause of death. A sensitive ME will understand a family's attempt to hide the facts. Likewise, hunting accidents involving one person are most likely suicides.

Some other signs can support suicide as cause of death. For example, if a right-handed person shoots himself in the torso with a long gun, usually the bullet has a downward, left-to-right trajectory. Conversely, when a left-handed person shoots himself in the body with a long gun, the bullet will follow a downward, right-to-left path. People who kill themselves also typically move aside any clothing before pulling the trigger.

Bullet fragments can also help a medical examiner determine if a gunshot victim was a suicide or a homicide. Invisible to the naked eye, these microscopic pieces of fired bullet can be embedded in the victim's clothes or skin. The fragments show up on X-rays of each bullet wound—done before the victim's clothes are removed. A fragment pattern can indicate the distance from which the shot was fired—and if it was even possible for the victim to shoot herself. If the ME or ballistics expert finds the shot was fired from a distance inconsistent with suicide dynamics, the death is ruled an accident or a homicide.

The gun will be examined for fingerprints and the hands for traces of gunpowder as well as fragments of hair, bone, and tissue. Bullet splatter will also likely be found on the hands or sleeves of suicide shooting victims.

Another common method of suicide is hanging, often with a rope. A person can die in one of three ways from hanging: strangulation, a broken neck, or—in extreme cases—decapitation. To hang himself, the suicide victim often ties a slip knot, makes a noose, loops it over his head, and turns it so the knot rests at the back or side of his neck. This type of knot tightens easily when the person suspends himself from a tree branch outdoors or a beam in a building, for example. Placement of the knot also has an effect on vertebra displacement—in judicial hangings, placing the knot under the left ear is often recommended, although some report that placement of the knot under the chin is more effective in dislocating the neck (Hellier and Connolly 2009).

A short drop can mean a comparatively slow death by strangulation, as a person dangles and finally loses consciousness after a minute or two. The taut rope around the person's neck makes breathing impossible and prevents blood from flowing through the carotid arteries. As the person dies, he experiences hypoxemia (a lack of oxygen in the blood), hypercarbia (increased blood levels of carbon dioxide), and acidosis (an increase in blood acidity). His brain may become herniated and swell. If he struggles—as is likely in this case—his heart rate rises and increases the amount of carbon dioxide in his blood.

Meanwhile, blood vessels rupture in the person's face and neck above the compressed noose, and blood is forced into tissues, creating ecchymosis (bruising). The skin and mucous membranes may develop a blue tint, indicating pressure on the jugular veins and a lack of oxygen. The victim's tongue may look enlarged, while petechiae (small ruptured blood vessels in the eyes) may appear (Wecht 2004). Pressure on the neck may also damage the carotid arteries, creating a vaso-vagal cardiac disruption and unconsciousness—in about six seconds (Hellier and Connolly 2009).

Hanging victims apparently suffer less when their necks are broken or dislocated—often a goal of judicial hangings. The drop distance needed to break a neck depends on the person's body mass; typically a distance between five feet and nine feet will do. The hanged person's neck breaks when his falling body reaches the end of the rope, rapidly tightens the noose, and wrenches his neck sideways, dislocating or snapping his neck's axis bone. The broken axis bone will likely sever the spinal cord, creating spinal shock and plunging blood pressure, so that the hanged person loses consciousness within seconds. His brain dies within a few minutes; complete death usually takes up to twenty minutes longer.

However, too long a drop (again, depending on the person's body mass) means too much force will be exerted on the victim's neck when he reaches the end of the rope. This results in the person's head coming off. Decapitation is more likely with a heavy person and a ligature made from a somewhat inelastic material, such as plastic-covered wire or nylon rope. In very rare circumstances, suicidal decapitations have occurred when the victim attaches a rope between his neck and a solid, stationary object, gets in his car and steps on the gas (Byard and Gilbert 2004).

A hanging victim who was not decapitated will have a particular mark: an inverted V-shaped furrow around his neck, following the path of the rope (or other ligature), slanting upward toward the knot. At this point, the furrows on either side of the neck should taper out to where the knot extended outward from the skin. The furrow will be white with a reddish rim right after death. If the body is left hanging, this rim will turn brown. If the victim does not have a V-shaped furrow around his neck, he probably did not die from hanging. Rather, a furrow that wraps around the neck without the V-shape indicates that strangulation—without suspension—may have been the cause of death.

However, someone who dies during autoerotic asphyxia, presumably hanging himself accidentally during this extreme activity, will usually not have a furrow in his neck. People who practice this activity typically use padding, such as towels, between the ligature and their necks to avoid leaving marks. Sometimes someone who dies this way has his hands tied or handcuffed. The medical examiner then must determine if this person was capable of hanging himself with his hands restrained. If not, of course, the death can no longer be considered an accident or a suicide.

In June 2009, actor David Carradine's death in Thailand sparked plenty of media speculation that he had accidentally killed himself during an autoerotic act. Reports emerged that the seventy-two-year-old was found nude with cords wrapped around his wrists, neck, and genitals. Thai police initially said they suspected the death was a suicide, but after conflicting reports, Carradine's family hired forensic pathologist Michael Baden for a private autopsy. Baden ruled out suicide, but at this book's writing, the police and forensic investigations were ongoing. While Baden ruled the cause of death was asphyxiation—an inability to breathe—manner of death at this book's writing was yet undetermined (Donaldson James 2009; Itzkoff 2009; Soonprasert 2009).

As at other types of death scenes, medical examiners sometimes need additional forensic expertise in suspected suicide cases. In the following case, the ME relied on a botanist and forensic anthropologists to determine if a hanging victim committed suicide or was murdered. In October 1990, a man found a human skeleton in Withlacoochee State Park in Pinellas County, Florida. Most of the bones lay on the ground below a tree, along with a man's clothing, some black electrician's tape, two knives, a piece of fabric, and a set of swimmer's goggles with electrician's tape covering the lens. About thirty or forty feet above, a rope tied with a noose hung over the branch of a tree. A small neck bone was broken and caught in the noose.

During the investigation of this death, a botanist estimated that a plant growing around the rope was a year to two years old, indicating the victim had been hanging from the tree for as long as two years before most of the skeleton had fallen to the ground. Anthropologists Robert Mann and Doug Owsley studied the bones in a lab in Washington, D.C., and concluded the victim was a white male, thirty to thirty-five years old and approximately five feet nine inches tall. The victim's pants size and length suggested they would fit a man of this height.

Mann noted that three pieces of electrical tape were overlapped to form one large piece with a raised area in the middle, shaped like a nose, and that the tape had been placed over the victim's mouth. He surmised the goggles were on the victim's face when the tape was applied. Mann became increasingly convinced that he was looking at a victim of homicide, not suicide. In his and Owsley's opinion, the piece of fabric found at the scene was used as a gag or to bind the victim's hands or feet. Other signs pointed to foul play: long fractures in the victim's ribs indicated trauma shortly before or shortly after he was hanged. Had the injuries occurred months after death, the ribs would simply have snapped in two.

Pinellas County Police believed they knew the identity of the victim: Randall Andrews, a thirty-two-year-old drifter. So at Mann and Owsley's request an FBI computer expert superimposed Andrews's photograph over an image of the victim's skull. The two images fit perfectly. To confirm the findings, an FBI forensic odontologist positively matched teeth found at the death scene with Andrews's dental records and X-rays.

Informants told police that several men beat and killed Andrews after he came across a farm where marijuana was grown. Police made arrests and pressed charges, but had insufficient evidence to try the suspects (Mann and Williamson 2006).

The deaths—even suicides—of movie stars and other public figures can spawn seemingly endless speculation. Conspiracy theorists and sensationalist tabloid reporters in particular won't let some celebrities rest in peace—especially when some of the facts aren't so clear-cut. Few of the famous, or infamous, continue to attract more ongoing interest than actress Marilyn Monroe. Here are some agreed-upon specifics regarding her death.

Monroe, who was born out of wedlock, lived in eleven foster homes while growing up. Her career was a success, but she was a lonely and insecure woman with psychiatric problems that included depression. For years she took sleeping pills and the water-soluble sedative chloral hydrate. Monroe also took Nembutal (pentobarbital sodium), a short-acting barbiturate used to treat insomnia, seizures, and convulsions. Long before the events directly leading to her death, Monroe had already overdosed on this drug and had been resuscitated.

In August 1962, at the insistence of her psychiatrist, Dr. Ralph Greenson, Monroe hired a live-in psychiatric nurse/housekeeper, Eunice K. Murray, to watch over her at her rented house in Brentwood. On the morning of Saturday, August 4, 1962, Monroe was in good spirits during breakfast. Suddenly she asked Murray if there was oxygen in the house. Murray replied no, and asked Monroe why she inquired about oxygen; Monroe said she was curious. At noon, Monroe had an argument with Pat Newcomb, her friend and press agent, who had slept over the night before and had removed her sleeping pills.

In the afternoon, Dr. Greenson arrived. Murray had telephoned him about Monroe's question regarding oxygen. He spent two hours with the actress and later described her as confused and disoriented. At 7:30 P.M., she was laughing and talking on the telephone with Joe DiMaggio, Jr., son of her ex-husband, baseball legend Joe DiMaggio, whom she had married and divorced in 1954.

Around midnight, Murray woke up and noticed the light was on in Monroe's bedroom. It was not like Monroe to have the light on that late. The door was locked; Monroe did not respond when Murray called out to her. Murray telephoned Dr. Greenson, who rushed over shortly after midnight and used a poker from the fireplace to break into the bedroom.

Monroe lay motionless and nude on her bed, her arm outstretched, her hand on the telephone. Bottles of pills, including chloral hydrate and a bottle of Nembutal—missing forty capsules—cluttered the bedside table. They found no note. Her physician, Dr. Hyman Engelberg, arrived and checked her heart with a stethoscope, examined her pupils, and pronounced her dead. Monroe was thirty-six years old.

Engelberg had recently prescribed fifty Nembutal for Monroe; she'd had the prescription filled Friday, August 3.

At 4:25 A.M., nearly four hours after Monroe's death. Greenson telephoned the West Los Angeles police station. Sgt. Jack Clemmons, who responded to the death scene, doubted Greenson and Murray's explanation that they spent four hours on the telephone talking to some of Monroe's business associates and movie studio contacts before calling police. Although he was not a detective, Clemmons suspected Monroe's body had been positioned and the death scene altered. In his opinion, Monroe was murdered.

Dr. Thomas T. Noguchi conducted Monroe's autopsy. During the external examination, he used a hand-held magnifying glass to check for needle marks. Any such marks would suggest Monroe had either injected herself—or been injected—with drugs. Noguchi did not find any of these telltale marks.

However, on her lower left back just above her hip, he found an ecchymosis—a type of bruise made when blood vessels rupture and leak blood into the surrounding tissues. The dark reddish blue color indicated the bruise was fresh. Noguchi could not account for this mark.

During the internal examination, Noguchi could not see any evidence of pills in Monroe's stomach or small intestine, nor any residue—although her stomach and gastric lining were reddened, a standard for barbiturate abuse. The lack of residue in Monroe's stomach didn't surprise Noguchi. Like the liver, the stomach gets used to the drug and rapidly passes it to the small intestine.

Toxicological analysis revealed Monroe's blood contained 8 mg of chloral hydrate and her liver, 13 mg of Nembutal. Her blood levels alone were the equivalent to forty or fifty regular-strength sleeping pills. For most people, ten to fifteen pills are deadly.

Although Noguchi wanted to send some of Monroe's other body fluids and organs, including her urine and a kidney, for further toxicological study, head toxicologist Raymond J. Abernathy apparently felt this was unnecessary. Based on Noguchi's autopsy and other evidence, Los Angeles Chief Medical Examiner Dr. Theodore J. Curphey concluded that Monroe died from an overdose of Nembutal and chloral hydrate pills. Manner of death: probable suicide.

Others have made different conclusions, particularly as the actress had connections with powerful men. Monroe had attended parties at the Santa Monica home of actor Peter Lawford, the brother-in-law of President John F. Kennedy. The president's brother, Attorney General Robert F. Kennedy, also attended parties at Lawford's house. Monroe has been linked romantically to both men.

Monroe apparently had learned some sensitive political information from the president about the Cold War, including information about nuclear weapons. Some believe she was considered a threat to the government after her involvement with the Kennedy brothers ended. Just weeks before her death, she telephoned Robert Kennedy eight times at the Justice Department.

On the evening of her death, Monroe refused an invitation from Lawford to attend a party at his house. Furthermore, she was found in the nude—rare for women who commit suicide. By 1982, continuing public fascination with Monroe's death led to an official investigation by the

Los Angeles District Attorney's Office into allegations of a conspiracy and cover-up. Mike Carroll, the former district attorney in charge of the investigation, concluded there was no evidence of an intentional criminal act concerning her death—although he noted contradictory statements from witnesses. To this day, the death of Marilyn Monroe continues to intrigue and puzzle her fans who wonder: suicide or murder? (The Marilyn 2006; Noguchi and DiMona 1983).

Another case that generated theories of murder and cover-ups is that of Robert Maxwell. In November 1991, the sixty-eight-year-old Maxwell was cruising on his 180-foot yacht, *Ghislaine*, near Grand Canary Island off the west coast of Africa. Maxwell, a Holocaust survivor and billionaire publishing magnate, had taken to his yacht to cure a cold he'd had for some time. Eleven crew members were aboard.

Maxwell, born Ludvik Hoch in Solotvino, Czechoslovakia, was a Jew whose parents, brother, three sisters, and grandparents died during the Holocaust. He escaped to England, joined the British Army, and became a captain. After working for British intelligence in Berlin, he returned to England in 1947. In 1964, as a Labor Party candidate, he won a seat in the House of Commons.

At approximately 5 A.M. on November 4, 1991, he called the bridge to say his stateroom was too cold. Later, when he did not answer a call, his staff began searching for him. He had left the stateroom, locked the door, and—apparently unseen by anyone—either fell, jumped, or was pushed to his death. About twelve hours after Maxwell called the bridge, a rescuer in a Spanish helicopter spotted Maxwell's naked 350-pound body floating face up in the waters off Grand Canary Island. Maxwell was taken to Tenerife, the largest of the seven Canary Islands belonging to Spain, where three pathologists performed the autopsy.

The pathologists found a graze on the forehead and a cut behind the ear, as well as bruising consistent with the rescue. They found no evidence of any violence that could have killed him, and he had no marks on his body to indicate suicide. The pathologists determined the manner of death was accidental. Respiratory cardiac arrest was noted as the cause of death on his death certificate.

According to British pathologists, however, respiratory cardiac arrest is not a cause of death. It's a mechanism of death; a way a person can die. Myocardial infarction or coronary thrombosis on the certificate would indicate a heart attack, but this was not mentioned.

Dr. Joseph Joseph, Maxwell's private doctor, suggested the death was suspicious. Maxwell's body was transported to Israel, where Dr. Iain West, one of Britain's leading pathologists, was sent by the Lloyds group of insurance companies to perform an autopsy on Maxwell. Suicide as manner of death would void the insurance payment to Maxwell's family.

During the autopsy, West worked with his wife, a pathologist, as well as three Israeli pathologists. It was a challenging assignment, as Maxwell's body had already been autopsied and embalmed. For example, the pathologists were uncertain who or what caused the abrasion on Maxwell's corpse— air-sea rescuers, Spanish pathologists, or the embalmer.

All the same, West challenged the findings of the Spanish pathologists. He believed Maxwell's left hand was injured and his left shoulder muscles torn while he was clinging to something—possibly a yacht railing. Like the Spanish pathologists, West did not find water in Maxwell's lungs—indicating the billionaire did not drown. While in West's opinion Maxwell's injuries did not rule out suicide, the pathologist also suggested that Maxwell may have had a seizure, fallen overboard, and been injured while trying to save himself. West concluded that if Maxwell had had a heart attack, he would have fallen onto the deck and could not have fallen into the sea. Yet the pathologist was unable to determine the exact cause of death.

Insurance companies supported the view that Maxwell had committed suicide, for the following reasons: he was in financial crisis; he had an uncommonly pleasant manner when dealing with others prior to his death; he kept to himself while aboard the yacht; his bedroom cabin was locked after Maxwell went on deck; and the key to the cabin was missing after his death. However, theories circulated about Maxwell's death, including that he laundered money; the Mossad murdered him; he was a gun runner; and the CIA killed him (Bower 1992; Thomas and Dillon 2002).

One last case created controversy due to the victim's high political connections—and because a few details of his death are not certain. On July 20, 1993, Deputy White House Counsel Vincent W. Foster Jr. drove six-and-a-half miles from Washington, D.C., to Fort Marcy in suburban Virginia. Foster, a friend of President Bill Clinton and First Lady Hillary Clinton, and formerly a law partner of Mrs. Clinton, then died of a gunshot wound—apparently self-inflicted.

A private citizen found Foster's body by a cannon near Chain Bridge Road and asked two off-duty Park Service employees to call 911. Park police and rescue personnel arrived shortly after 6 P.M. Foster lay on his back, a Colt Army Special .38 revolver in his right hand, his thumb trapped in the trigger guard. Material resembling gunshot residue marked that same hand. The revolver had a four-inch barrel and contained one live Remington round and one spent Remington casing. Police and Fairfax County Fire and Rescue Department (FCFRD) personnel searched the park, but the fatal bullet was not recovered. Its trajectory may have sent it over the trees and outside the park, or it may have ricocheted off an obstruction. The exterior surface of the revolver, meanwhile, was textured and not suitable for the formation of fingerprints, and so none would be found.

Later that evening, park police would turn over the body and find an exit wound on the back of Foster's head. Blood had pooled on the ground under his head and back. Investigators could find no sign of a struggle at the death scene, nor any indication that Foster had been dragged. Police found a

Honda Accord with Arkansas plates registered to Foster in the Fort Marcy parking lot. Some investigators at the death scene reported that a briefcase was in Foster's Honda; other investigators disagreed.

At about 7:40 P.M., medical examiner representative Dr. Donald Haut arrived and pronounced Foster dead. FCFRD ambulance personnel then drove Foster's body to the morgue at Fairfax Hospital in Fairfax, Virginia.

The next day Dr. James Beyer, deputy chief medical examiner of the Virginia Office of the Chief Medical Examiner, performed the autopsy. Beyer noted an entrance wound in the back of the mouth, a wound in the soft palate tissue, and powder debris in the soft palate and at the back of the mouth. The exit wound, irregular in shape and three inches from the top of the head, was one-and-one-quarter inches by one inch in size. The muzzle of the weapon had to have been in Foster's mouth, close to the back of his throat.

Beyer observed that there was much less gunpowder debris on Foster's left hand than on his right. An indentation mark on the inside of the right thumb was produced by the trigger of the .38. He found no evidence of trauma to the body other than the gunshot wound. He could not identify the food in Foster's stomach, but he saw nothing in Foster's central nervous system or any sort of disease that would have impeded Foster in preventing someone from placing a gun in his mouth and pulling the trigger. In addition, DNA consistent with Foster's was detected on the revolver's muzzle. X-rays were not taken, however, because even though the X-ray machine was new, it was not functioning. Dr. Beyer concluded that Foster's manner of the death was suicide.

The Office of Independent Counsel (OIC) retained experts to review this high-profile death. These included Dr. Brian D. Blackbourne, medical examiner of San Diego County, California; Dr. Henry C. Lee, director of the Connecticut State Police Forensic Science Laboratory; and Dr. Alan L. Berman, executive director of the American Association of Suicidology. All of the experts agreed with Beyer: Foster had committed suicide.

But a rumor circulated that Foster did not commit suicide because the revolver found in his hand was not his gun. Investigators spoke with Foster's family and established that, shortly before his death, Foster took possession of a number of guns that belonged to his father. Lisa Foster, Vincent Foster's wife, said that the revolver found at the death scene was the gun that was missing from the firearms her husband had received from his father. She said he had stored it at her and her husband's home.

At the time of his death, Foster was handling personal legal matters for the Clintons. The Clintons were involved with the Whitewater Development Corp., an Arkansas land venture, and Guaranty Savings and Loan Association, a business failure owned by Clinton friends James and Susan McDougal. Foster's connection with the presidential couple inspired yet another rumor—this time of a White House cover-up regarding his death.

Yet four days before his death, Foster told his sister he was depressed. The day before his death, he called his family doctor in Arkansas about anti-depressant medication. The doctor, Larry Watkins, prescribed trazodone (Desyrel) 50 mg. Foster's wife, Lisa, said that from July 16 to 18, Foster was considering resigning from work. However, if Foster left a suicide note, no one brought it forward.

The U.S. Court of Appeals for the District of Columbia released a report on Foster in October 1997. Written by independent counsel Kenneth W. Starr, the report noted that Foster was clinically depressed prior to his death and that days before his suicide, Foster had written that he was not suited to his job nor to the spotlight associated with public life in Washington (Whitewater 1998).

Some probable suicide cases will always generate controversy, while others may seem obvious right away. It's essential for medical examiners to avoid making snap judgments and to approach each death with an open mind.

8

———•◦•———

AUTOPSY SUITE AND EXAMINATION RESOURCES

MEDICAL EXAMINERS' OFFICES tend to have more similarities than differences due to the nature of the work and the necessary equipment. To give readers a sense of these facilities, the following is an illustration of a medical examiner's office, drawn from several ME offices in widespread communities.

In this typical ME office, employees arrive at a front entrance. The doors are controlled electronically, and security cameras watch over everyone who arrives and departs. To the left of the entrance is the reception area foyer, where police officers, the family of a decedent, and reporters wait for news—or to view a body. Just past them are offices for administrative staff. A hallway stretches off the reception area, with seminar rooms and washrooms opening on either side and ending at the library entrance. Most of the library resources are about causes of death and death investigations. They include books, periodicals, CDs, DVDs, and databases.

Next to the library is a common room with counters, tables, chairs, refrigerator, microwave ovens, water fountain, and soft drink machine. Another hallway extends past the library to double doors marked with the words "Restricted Area." Staff members with access use a key card to unlock the doors. Once through, they see the toxicology lab on the left side of the hallway, and farther on, the family room on the right.

In the family room, grief counselors accompany people who must identify the dead body of someone they know, perhaps a relative or a friend. This room is dimly lit and, like other rooms throughout the ME facility, is spotlessly clean and painted in subdued colors. The room has the low-key feel of a living room thanks to its furnishings—a sofa, several chairs, a couple of end tables, and one or two lamps. One wall may have a discreet, soft-hued painting; the other wall is hung with drapes. Behind the drapes is a window. When the drapes are parted, the people in the room will see part of a walk-in cooler.

This cooler contains wall units with large pullout drawers for bodies, which may be stored there from a few days to weeks. The wall units keep the bodies cool. The temperature is low—about 40 degrees Fahrenheit. This keeps in-house decomposition at a relatively slow rate. The deceased's family and friends cannot see the shelves that line one of the cooler room's walls. Hidden from public view, these shelves house dozens of bodies, including corpses that must wait long periods of time to be identified. Also blocked from the sight of visitors is the decomposition room as well as shelves that contain hundreds of jars of organ tissue and brains in preservative. The decomposition room, an adjacent cooler, is used to store severely decayed bodies before they are autopsied.

There are three ways a person in the family room may identify a decedent. First, a pathology assistant wheels the body on a metal gurney to the window and slowly pulls down a clean white sheet to reveal the face. Second, the deceased person on the gurney is positioned under a camera near the drawer where the body was stored, and then a person in the family room views the decedent's face on a television monitor opposite the window. Third, a pathology assistant walks to the window and holds a black-and-white Polaroid photograph of the decedent close to the window. The ME and pathology assistant consider the body's condition before choosing an option. A black-and-white photograph of a dead person with a disfigured face, covered with makeup, is probably less traumatic for a caring family to view.

The grief counselor may step out of the room for a few minutes while the family or friends react to identifying the body. Sometimes, like family or friends at a death scene, they will become angry and vent their anger on the counselor. A security guard or police officer may have to intervene in extreme cases of aggression and violence.

The door to the autopsy suite is inside the walk-in cooler. Once within, shining white tile and gleaming stainless steel dominate. The lighting is bright, and at each autopsy station, a slightly tilted, stainless steel dissection table reclines. Water runs along the length of the two inside edges of each table and washes body fluids toward an attached sink. Containers with preservative for storing organs are handy, and the ME's autopsy instruments are neatly arranged near the dissection table. Biohazard bags are nearby to dispose of tissue that is not kept or washed down the sink. The bags will be incinerated after an autopsy. A stepladder is stored close by for the photographer to use when she is photographing a body from above. A radio or CD player plays music.

Safety equipment is paramount among an ME's examination resources. The autopsy suite is well stocked with essential protective gear. Everyone at an autopsy should wear a surgical scrub suit, surgical cap, long-sleeved gown, apron, goggles or face shield, shoe covers, and double surgical gloves. An N-95 respirator, masklike in appearance, is preferred to a surgical mask because the respirator's fabric is much more likely to filter out an airborne contaminant such as *M. tuberculosis* (TB). An ME may wear powered air-purifying respirators (PAPRs) equipped with N-95 or high-efficiency particulate air (HEPA) cartridge filters, as opposed to using only an N 95 respirator. The ME may have disposable N-95 and HEPA respirators on hand. These protect the eyes, skin, and mucous membranes from blood-borne and aerosol transmissible pathogens (Nolte, Taylor, and Richmond 2002).

Cleanliness and proper safety precautions are critical at the ME's office. Medical examiners and other professionals at an autopsy are also wary of infectious agents that may infect them in a cut or scratch. These microorganisms invade body tissues and multiply, injuring the host's cells because of an antigen-antibody response or replication between cells. Antigens stimulate an immune response because the immune system recognizes them as foreign substances in the body and then produces antibodies, protein substances that destroy or neutralize bacteria, viruses, or other harmful toxins. Infectious agents may be defeated if the body's defense mechanisms are effective. However, a local infection may spread when the microorganisms gain access to the lymphatic system, the tissues and organs that produce and store cells that fight infection and disease.

Medical examiners can become injured and infected with microorganisms by cutting themselves with contaminated needles, scalpels, embedded needle fragments, bone shards, and fragmented projectiles. People who die from AIDS, tuberculosis, diphtheria, hepatitis B, or hepatitis C are a potential source of infections that can be passed to medical examiners who accidentally cut themselves while performing autopsies.

At some medical examiner offices, staff put a sign or label on a body to clearly identify the deceased as having a specific infectious condition, indicating that the person is a high-risk autopsy. There is a very high correlation in some areas of the U.S. between hepatitis C virus (HCV) and decedents who abused drugs intravenously. This poses a serious health threat to MEs who perform their autopsies.

Corpses infected with HIV are considered infectious for at least two weeks after death. Hepatitis B virus (HBV) in human plasma, the clear, yellowish fluid portion of blood, lymph, or intra-muscular fluid in which cells are suspended, may be infectious a week after being dried and exposed to an ambient environment. Medical examiners have died of diseases transmitted by cuts to the skin during autopsies, including Marburg, Ebola, and Lassa hemorrhagic fevers.

A medical examiner can also become ill from inhaling infectious aerosols, airborne particles that can remain suspended in the air for long periods of time. After these particles are inhaled, they cross the upper respiratory passages and access the body tissues through the pulmonary alveoli, tiny, thin-walled, air-filled sacs in the lungs. Some particles may become airborne because of the action of the fluid aspirator hoses venting into the sinks, the oscillating saws that cut bones and soft tissues, or water sprayed from hoses onto tissue surfaces. Droplets or larger particles have less potential to travel the distances beyond the autopsy area. But an autopsy can efficiently spread, in as brief a time as ten minutes, TB from the cadaver to everyone present in the suite.

It has happened. The Syracuse Medical Examiner's Office and the Los Angeles Coroner's Office experienced outbreaks of autopsy-transmitted tuberculosis, due to inadequate ventilation, in the 1990s (Nolte, Taylor, and Richmond 2002).

Prions are another serious risk to medical examiners during autopsy. The word *prion* stands for "proteinaceous infectious pathogen" and was coined by Stanley Prusiner, an American neurologist and 1997 Nobel Prize winner. These infectious agents attack the central nervous system by altering protein in the brain so that brain cells deteriorate, function abnormally, and die. Prions are associated with CJD (Creutzfeldt-Jakob Disease), a fatal disease named after German psychiatrists Hans G. Creutzfeldt (1883–1964) and Alfons M. Jakob (1884–1931), who independently described this disease during the first part of the twentieth century.

CJD is the human variant of mad cow disease occasionally detected in cattle native to the U.S. or in cattle shipped from Canada to the U.S. and used for human consumption. The symptoms of CJD include weight loss, loss of sexual drive, blurry vision, disorientation, hallucinations, muscle spasms, and difficulty moving. A person with this fatal disease can expect to live about a year from the onset of symptoms (Frankel 2005; Gale 2002; Prusiner 1984; Robinson 2002).

Although formalin, also known as formaldehyde solution, is an essential preservative and fixative for pathologic specimens, it does not deactivate prions. Prions can be transmitted even when they are encased in paraffin blocks—a method of tissue sample storage. These blocks, kept in small plastic cassettes, contain pieces of tissue that can be cut into very thin slices for study under a microscope. While useful, formaldehyde use poses its own risks. Formaldehyde is a toxic agent and can irritate eyes and mucous membranes. Signs of formaldehyde overexposure include watering eyes, difficulty breathing, a burning sensation in the throat, and headache. Long-term inhalation of formaldehyde has been associated with an increased risk of cancer.

MEs and their staff are also occasionally exposed to cyanide when they perform autopsies on people who ingested this chemical compound. This extremely toxic and fast-acting poison can evaporate from autopsy tissues and be inhaled, but a greater risk occurs when the ME opens a decedent's stomach. Cyanide salts are converted to highly volatile hydro-cyanic gas in the stomach. For this reason, the stomach should be opened in a completely exhausted bio-safety cabinet, or under a chemical fume hood, if a medical examiner wants to avoid inhaling potentially toxic concentrations of this gas.

Medical examiners without proper safety precautions can also get headaches and become nauseous after opening the stomachs of people who consumed fatal doses of metallic phosphides used in pellets for killing rodents.

Phosphides and stomach acids form phosphine, a colorless, flammable gas that is highly poisonous and is fatal in relatively low concentrations. Medical examiners should wear gloves when handling potentially contaminated personal articles of decedents who died of organophosphate pesticide poisoning.

Forensic pathologists may encounter other serious threats while performing their duties in the autopsy suite. Nerve gas agents such as sarin and soman are chemical war and bioterrorism weapons that can slowly penetrate heavy rubber gloves and aprons and be absorbed through the skin. Decedents contaminated with these agents should be washed, preferably with an alkaline solution, possibly 5 percent hypochlorite, a disinfectant containing chlorine. A self-contained breathing apparatus (SCBA), similar to the type used by firefighters, should be mandatory for medical examiners in case of these dangerous nerve gas agents (Nolte, Taylor, and Richmond 2002).

As mentioned in Chapter 6, autopsies are sometimes performed on people whose bodies contain radioactive materials, often from diagnostic or therapeutic procedures. Without adequate precautions, the ME can be exposed to excessive radiation when she performs an autopsy on a person who recently underwent a gallium scan, a nuclear medicine procedure used to detect areas of infection or rapid cell division in the body, as in cancer. A body containing an isotope that has a long half-life—for example, strontium-90 (twenty-eight years)—may be better buried than autopsied (Nolte, Taylor, and Richmond 2002).

Because of all these dangers, autopsy suites should be physically separate from other areas of the medical examiner's offices and be designed to prevent contaminated air from entering the rest of the medical examiner's offices. Administrative areas, for example, should have a separate air supply. Separation should ensure that only fully protected autopsy staff is exposed to blood-borne and aerosolized pathogens.

Ideally, air in autopsy suites is exchanged at least twelve times per hour and should be under negative pressure in relation to surrounding spaces. Negative pressure—or pressure less than that of the ambient atmosphere—causes air to flow into the room from the outside whenever a door is opened. The air in autopsy suites should flow in one direction: from clean areas to potentially contaminated areas. This air should then be exhausted directly to the outside of the medical examiner facility. Other features to help decrease the exposure of autopsy room staff to airborne pathogens include downdraft autopsy tables, ultraviolet irradiation devices for sterilizing air, HEPA filters, and biological safety cabinets for handling infected tissues (al-Wali, Kibbler, and McLaughlin 1993; Martin, Nemitz, Hendley, Fisk, and Wells 1995; Nolte, Taylor, and Richmond 2002).

Another examination resource that must be handled with care is toluidine blue, a dye that may cause eye and skin irritation. This dye is used to detect genital and anal injuries invisible to the naked eye, typically in sexual assault cases on live and dead victims. Toluidine blue does not stain skin that is intact, but a stain remains on areas with trauma, such as on an abrasion. The ME or pathology assistant takes color photographs before and after toluidine blue is applied (Geberth 2003; Hochmeister, Whelan, Borer, Gehrig, Binda, Berzianovich, Rauch, and Dirnhofer 1997). The medical examiner uses cotton or gauze to apply toluidine blue to an area where there is suspected trauma. She will use K-Y jelly, a water-based personal lubricant, or a similar substance to remove excess toluidine blue, as this lubricant does not contain color or perfume additives, does not stain, and is easy to clean up.

Another autopsy room resource is the Wood's lamp, invented in 1903 by Baltimore, Maryland, physicist Robert W. Wood, who first used it to detect ringworm of the scalp. Today the Wood's lamp is used as a handheld alternate light source about the size of a large flashlight and is used in darkness, with orange goggles, to detect organic material invisible to the naked eye.

Most body fluids, including semen, fluoresce in the violet and blue spectrums—although saliva and blood do not show this effect. To detect semen, the medical examiner dons the goggles, turns on the Wood's lamp, and directs blue light over the person's clothes and body. When detected, semen appears as an irregular orange splotch (Baden and Roach 2001; Cataldie 2006).

On the subject of light, a standard resource in the autopsy suite is a light box illuminated by fluorescent bulbs. This is where the medical examiner views X-rays and can spot telling details. For example, the light box will make a bullet in a skull readily visible as the bullet contrasts with the bone. This is one way for the ME to determine where the bullet stopped after entering the head—alternatively, she may insert a probe into the wound channel.

One newer resource is the ability to isolate DNA and its arrangement on each chromosome, thereby creating a profile of the decedent's individual genetic code. Each person's DNA in, for example, every skin cell or every bone cell, is unique with the exception of identical twins.

DNA fingerprinting, also known as DNA typing and DNA profiling, is a lab procedure that uses DNA to identify people, including perpetrators. To create a DNA fingerprint, a sample is taken from body tissue or a fluid such as blood. Chewing gum, bandages, and drinking cups are other sources of DNA. Enzymes, proteins that speed up chemical reactions in living organisms, divide the DNA sample into smaller components. DNA is further divided by electrophoresis, the motion of charged particles in a colloid under the influence of an electric field. A colloid is a mixture of undissolved particles that do not settle in the mixture. After the segments are marked and exposed on X-ray film, they form a pattern of black bars that constitute the DNA fingerprint.

Next, blood, saliva, and semen—or other DNA-rich samples from death scenes—are compared with samples obtained from perpetrators, persons of interest, or family members. This is usually done in suspicious death cases or when the decedent needs to be identified. Comparisons can link a person to or eliminate him from a crime scene; they can also identify decedents who died in mass disasters. Forensic scientists and police labs use DNA fingerprinting as evidence in criminal proceedings.

Acquiring DNA for testing can be tricky—often permission or a court order is needed in suspicious death cases. Sometimes, during the questioning of a suspect, police will offer the suspect a cigarette. After the suspect leaves the room, police will retrieve the cigarette butt from an ashtray and use the saliva on the butt for DNA testing. The suspect's DNA can be compared at the medical examiner's office to DNA found on a John or Jane Doe homicide victim to determine if the suspect's DNA is on the victim, thus establishing a link between suspect and victim (*American College* 2003; Baden and Roach 2001; Chabner 2004).

DNA comparisons are done with the help of the Combined DNA Index System (CODIS), a computer network connecting forensic DNA labs throughout the U.S. Every state has agreed to establish a DNA database to retain DNA profiles of offenders convicted of violent crimes. CODIS has local, state, and national tiers, or levels. All three tiers contain forensic and convicted offender information, as well as a population file used to generate statistics.

This electronic resource helps medical examiners link the Jane or John Doe homicide victims in their coolers with offenders convicted of homicide and other crimes, if unknown DNA on a body can be matched to the DNA of a convicted offender. This DNA may be from sperm: some perpetrators of sexually related homicide masturbate on or near their victims, leaving behind their DNA signatures. Matching this DNA to records in CODIS establishes a link between a known perpetrator and the deceased.

Different CODIS indexes can be searched. The convicted offender index contains DNA profiles of individuals convicted of a variety of crimes, including sexual assault and murder. Criteria for deciding which offenders must submit DNA vary from state to state. The forensic index has DNA profiles obtained from crime scene evidence—for example, semen and blood. The missing persons index includes the unidentified persons index and the reference index. The unidentified persons index contains DNA profiles from recovered remains: bone, teeth, and hair. The reference index has DNA profiles of relatives of missing persons so these profiles can periodically be compared to the unidentified persons index (Becker 2005).

Some medical examiners have access to CALGANG, a database with information about gang members in California. Information categories include characteristics of gang tattoos, among others. Such a marking could help provide clues to a dead person's identity when compared to information about tattoos in CALGANG. The Florida Department of Law Enforcement had a similar idea in 2004 when it developed a database containing information on more than 372,000 tattoos on state prisoners.

The autopsy suite is a place of extremes, both a lively workplace and a destination for the dead. Bodies arrive under a veil of mystery, yet their identities and causes of death may soon be discovered. Ultimately, the autopsy suite is a place where the medical examiner works toward truth and justice.

9

AUTOPSY: EXTERNAL EXAMINATION

THE MEDICAL DETECTIVE work begins from the moment the body bag is unsealed or the evidence sheet is pulled away. That's unless, of course, the medical examiner observed the body at the death scene, an ideal not all jurisdictions can afford. In many forensic autopsies, the ME first meets the deceased on his worktable. This is the time when he can take a thorough look at the body before applying the scalpel or other equipment—and determine whether additional forensic experts need to be brought in.

Typically, the ME does not do the heavy lifting. The morgue attendant or diener, a German word for "servant," brings the body from the cooler to the autopsy suite. The diener may also assist during the autopsy and clean up the autopsy suite afterward.

The police officer or other authorized person who identified the body at the death scene should be present at the morgue or medical examiner's office. The officer witnesses the body being removed from the cooler, rolled into the autopsy suite, revealed within the body bag, photographed taken from the body bag, and placed on the autopsy table. He notes the time this is done. This witnessing process ensures a chain of custody—meaning that only authorized and documented people have had access to the body. If, for example, a body was considered evidence in a murder, a broken chain of custody could indicate evidence tampering and lead to a mistrial.

The officer next compares a death scene photo—or photo identification of the deceased—to the identification tag usually tied to the decedent's big toe. This helps ensure the body on the autopsy table is the same body that was at the death scene. A toe is a good place for the ID tag because it is usually not a significant location for forensic evidence; in addition, the toe is readily accessible when the body is in a body bag. This helps a medical examiner quickly confirm the decedent's identity. Other possible locations for the ID tag include the ankle or wrist (Koehler and Wecht 2006).

While the decedent is still fully clothed, the medical examiner photographs the body with a 35 millimeter camera, a Polaroid, a digital camera, or sometimes a combination of the three. This step records the position of the clothing, information that could become important in court cases. The medical examiner makes sure to include something in the photograph to give a sense of scale, typically a six-inch ruler, as well as an identification number. These photographs help establish the decedent's identity as well as show the person's injuries in relation to the condition of any clothing. Subsequent photographs will show the body in various stages of undress as the ME considers the position as well as the condition of the garments and correlates tears or other defects with visible injuries. To avoid flaws in his investigation, the ME keeps in mind that a number of perpetrators undress their victims after death and may replace some or all of the clothing.

Just as police officers are careful to watch out for needles when searching known drug addicts, the ME must also take care when handling the decedent's clothes. Needles or other sharp objects could be in a pocket or elsewhere on the deceased's person. A minor needle prick could result in the ME contracting AIDS (Acquired Immune Deficiency Syndrome) or another life-threatening illness such as hepatitis, an inflammatory disease of the liver.

The ME takes care to unbutton buttons and unzip zippers. He also avoids tearing or cutting the clothes while looking for brand names, laundry marks, stains, clothing size, stab wounds, or bullet holes. The ME records the condition of the clothing so that all the evidence is accounted for if the body is involved in a criminal case. In a homicide case, for example, the defense could try to attribute a missing button to the autopsy, when in fact the button may have gone missing during the perpetrator's attack on the victim.

The medical examiner then takes the garments to a nearby table, lays them out to further establish relationships between the decedent's wounds and fabric tears or other damage, and takes more photographs if needed. This part of the external examination helps him determine the position of the deceased at the time any injuries were received. He will consider questions such as whether the decedent was seated or standing. When the ME sees a body, it is usually in a horizontal, motionless position. But until death, most bodies are dynamic, moving entities, particularly the arms. Determining a shooting victim's stance at death, for example, can help establish the bullet trajectory as well as the positioning of the shooter. The ME next ensures each item of clothing is properly marked for identification as evidence and is stored in a locked room.

If a forensic entomologist (an expert on insects inhabiting decomposing bodies) is involved with the case and has collected specimens at the death scene, she should also be present when the body is removed from the body bag. This is especially important when the decedent has advanced decomposition and is infested with insects. A maggot-infested body must be autopsied very soon, as hungry larvae can consume key evidence within a few days.

The forensic entomologist will check the body bag thoroughly, looking for larvae or adult specimens that may be on the outer and inner surfaces. Temperature changes or the handling of the deceased may have spurred the bugs to crawl away from the body inside the bag. The entomologist collects and labels any insects or larvae that she finds, noting where on the body these specimens were found—in clothing areas such as pockets or folds, and in torn or decayed remnants. All of these areas may yield eggs, larvae, pupae, or adult insects.

Often, if the decedent's hands were bagged and taped to preserve potential trace evidence—such as cells or fibers—the entomologist will also check these bags for any insects. After the deceased's clothing is examined and removed, she photographs areas of the body where insects are concentrated.

Any seeds or plant materials found should be collected for analysis by a forensic botanist (an expert on plant material associated with corpses). The life stages of insects, as well as the various parts of plants, may reveal clues about the time or place of the person's death. For example, if a type of insect or plant is found on the deceased but is typically not found in the location of the death scene, then it's possible the decedent died elsewhere and was dumped at the scene (Haskell, Lord, and Byrd 2001).

Next the ME uses an X-ray and fluoroscope (an X-ray device used to examine deep structures) to look for bullets, bullet fragments, shell casings, broken knife blades, fractures, anatomic deformities, post-surgical scars, metal plates, screws, nails, or other features of interest on or inside the decedent. Depending on the protocol of the ME's office, the medical examiner may X-ray the body before it is undressed, possibly while it's still inside the body bag.

The medical examiner photographs, in close proximity to the decedent, any potential murder weapons recovered from the death scene. He ensures the weapons and body are in the same photograph, yet sufficiently distant from each other to prevent transfer of evidence—such as blood, hair, soil, or fiber—from the decedent to the weapon, or vice versa. Transfer of evidence can weaken the prosecution's case, as it allows the defense to argue that an unprofessional investigation caused cross-contamination, indicating that the prosecution's methods are questionable. In this situation, the defense could ask for a mistrial.

The last part of the external examination is a head-to-toe assessment of the unclothed body. In what is known as the basic description, the medical examiner usually states his observations about the decedent into a handheld recorder, sometimes held by the diener. Even if a recorder is not used, the diener fills out a form on the decedent's identifiers: race, sex, height, weight, hair color, eye color, and location and description of moles, tattoos, or birth-marks.

Mikhail Gorbachev, the leader of the Soviet Union from 1985 to 1991, made one type of birthmark famous: the port wine stain, which resembled drips of strawberry jam on the bald top of his head. This type of birthmark is commonly located on the face and upper trunk, on only one side of the body. Other common birthmarks include a strawberry mark, a soft, red, raised swelling resembling its namesake berry, usually found on the face or neck and often disappearing by age nine; café au lait spots, flat, tan to light brown patches; and the Mongolian spot, a blue or gray mark typically found on the buttocks or back of babies with deeper skin color.

After identifying these observable details, the medical examiner describes the deceased's state of health before death. He uses words such as "healthy," "well nourished," or "undernourished." Another term he may use to describe various parts of the body during this part of the examination—or during the internal examination—is "unremarkable." He combs the deceased's scalp and pubic hair to check for hair from another person, and then plucks hairs, including their roots, from the scalp, eyebrows, armpits, and pubic region. One of these plucked hairs may match a sample found on a suspect or something belonging to a suspect, providing a key link between this suspect and the deceased. As the scalp hair can hide head injuries such as a small-caliber bullet wound, the ME examines the entire scalp carefully, sometimes shaving areas with a razor.

If a forensic entomologist hasn't already done so, the ME checks the nose and eyes for insect activity or evidence that insects such as blowflies have laid their eggs there. He also examines the eyes for petechiae, pinpoint-like red spots commonly found in strangulation victims. He then takes a large syringe, sinks the needle into the corner of one of the decedent's eyes, and withdraws vitreous humor, the gel-like substance inside the eyeball. He repeats the action with the other eye. As potassium levels increase in vitreous humor after death, the medical examiner may determine time of death by measuring the rising levels of postmortem potassium (see Chapter 2). The procedure leaves the deceased's eyes looking sunken, however, so the ME injects saline solution into them to restore a relatively normal appearance. Otherwise, the decedent's eyes would look frightening at an open-casket funeral (Ribowsky and Shachtman 2006).

Sometimes one or both eyes of a decedent will bulge forward and have a prominent stare. Called exophthalmos, this condition is caused by swelling eye socket tissues and is more common in women. Often it's associated with hyperthyroidism (overactive thyroid) or hypothyroidism (underactive thyroid), although protruding eyes are also a symptom of other medical conditions such as an infection behind the eyes or a tumor (American College 2003). Along with the bulging eyes, the ME may notice a goiter in the deceased's neck. Caused by swelling in the thyroid gland, it can be barely noticeable or as large as a grapefruit.

On the subject of eyes, the ME will remove the deceased's corneas within a week of death if they are to be donated to an eye bank. Beforehand, he tapes gauze over the decedent's eyes. This keeps the lids shut to prevent the corneas from drying out until they're removed.

The medical examiner takes a close look at the decedent's face. Traces of powder on the deceased's lips may mean the person took a drug before death. Vomit may indicate a drug or another substance irritated the person's stomach. Semen in the mouth may point to a sexual component in the death. The ME uses unwaxed dental floss to remove traces of this body fluid from between teeth.

Moving down the body, the ME looks for more clues to what happened to the decedent. He may find defense wounds on the hands, wrists, and arms, suggesting the deceased attempted to fight off an attacker who used a knife or other sharp object, such as a broken bottle. Or the ME may notice defense wounds on the deceased's legs, even if the victim succeeded in kicking back at the perpetrator. These wounds can hide soil or shoe polish that's been transferred from attacker to victim—or vice versa—all useful clues in an investigation. He may note gunpowder on the hands if the decedent, perpetrator, or both fired at least one firearm. A person in close proximity to a shooter, however, may have gunpowder residue on his hands or clothes. The gun barrel emits gunpowder residue when the trigger is pulled; the closer the shooter is to the victim, the greater the amount of residue on the victim's clothes or skin.

The ME examines the hands and wrists for any unusual qualities or markings. Crack cocaine addicts may develop a callus on the palm-side surface of their thumbs by repeatedly flicking their cigarette lighters to keep the cocaine hot (Stephens, Jentzen, Karch, Mash, and Wetli 2004). Sometimes what's not there can provide clues as well. A sticky, hairless patch on the wrists, for example, may suggest a perpetrator used tape to bind the deceased. Bruising around twin areas of both wrists, meanwhile, is a sign the decedent may have been handcuffed. The ME examines the fingers. Healthy nails, usually a sign of a healthy person, are smooth and uniform in color. Mee's lines, bands of relatively parallel lines across the fingernails, indicate arsenic ingestion. If the deceased consumed any drugs or chemicals in the previous twelve months, toxicological tests may detect them in the nails—although the ME may prefer to check the big toenail for analysis as this nail is less likely to have been exposed to external contamination. Trace elements, including gold, copper, and silver, can also be detected in nails. The medical examiner clips the decedent's fingernails to check for minute amounts of fiber, pollen, human tissue, hair, glass fragments, or blood. Homicide victims who struggled with their killers sometimes have hair or tissue under their fingernails—leaving behind material useful for creating DNA profiles of their attackers (Daniel, Piraccini, and Tosti 2004; Litin 2003; New 2005; Palmeri, Pichini, Pacifici, Zuccaro, and Lopez 2000).

The medical examiner continues his scan of the body. He may note bite marks on the decedent's breasts, thighs, shoulders, or scrotum. He will try to recover any saliva from the bites to create a DNA profile of the perpetrator. A thorough medical examiner will also have a forensic dentist examine these marks.

The ME traces any gunshot or stab wounds from point of entry to point of termination or exit. Gunshot entrance wounds—as opposed to exit wounds—typically have an abrasion ring, an area around the wound where the bullet scraped the skin as it entered the body. Other signs of an entrance wound depend on the distance from which the bullet was shot. If he finds bullets or bullet fragments in a body, the medical examiner hands them over to homicide detectives, who in turn give them to the crime lab's ballistics expert. The ballistics expert knows about the movement and forces associated with the propulsion of objects through the air, including bullets.

The ME notes any non-penetrating injuries such as fractures (breaks) to bones and lacerations (tears) to blood vessels and tissue, and duly notes any mutilation, dismemberment, and, conversely, emergency medical treatment. Paramedics and hospital staff occasionally break ribs when they try to resuscitate an injured or sick person. Or, while trying to save a shooting or stabbing victim's life, they may have performed surgery or other procedures on wounds. Knowing about this kind of treatment before beginning the autopsy is essential for the ME. Any error in the autopsy report or the protocol not only reflects negatively on the medical examiner, it can have serious legal repercussions.

The medical examiner then takes nasal, oral, and rectal swabs—and vaginal swabs if the deceased is female—and sends the samples to a lab, particularly when sexual involvement is a suspected factor in the death (Geberth 1996; Genge 2002; Green 2000; Pounder 2000).

The ME is now ready to perform the internal autopsy.

10

AUTOPSY: INTERNAL EXAMINATION

MOST PEOPLE WHO end up on a medical examiner's table have died too soon: they've suffered violence, a terrible accident, or perished in an unexpected way. The person's family may be shocked and traumatized. But forensic pathologists must keep their feelings in check in order to do their job well. Often, medical examiners cultivate a sense of detached curiosity along with an open mind. Becoming emotionally involved with a case will do nothing to help solve the mysteries of the decedent's death.

Although a medical examiner's patient is no longer living, the ME usually reassures the decedent's family and friends that the deceased will be treated with dignity and respect. But autopsies aren't for the squeamish. While doctors who work with live patients must be careful not to inflict any bruises, it is inevitable that some damage will occur during an internal examination of a dead body—particularly if the body is already undergoing advanced decay processes. The body may also suffer some bumps during transportation or while being moved from body bag to table: skin may stick to the stainless steel dissection table or a less-experienced doctor may not yet have much finesse with a blade (Gawande 2001). None of this should interfere with the death investigation.

After completing the external examination, the medical examiner arranges the unclothed body face up on the autopsy table, and slides a rubber or plastic body block under the person's back. The chest protrudes upward, the arms and neck fall backward. This position allows the medical examiner best access to the trunk—the main part of the body. In some medical examiner offices, the diener (morgue assistant) performs some or all of these preliminary duties, but this depends on the administrative structure at a particular office.

The ME picks up a scalpel with a large, razor-sharp blade. The first cut she'll make is the Y-incision, also known as the thoracoabdominal incision. This incision can later be disguised by clothing so as not to be visible to relatives who may view the body. Like most doctors who perform surgery, the medical examiner will likely hold the scalpel with the thumb and four fingers, as though about to play a violin. This helps her slice through the skin at an even depth—about as deep as the rib cage, the curving bones that enclose the chest and protect the lungs, heart, and other internal organs (organs that perform functions essential to human life, such as the heart). She pierces the skin in front of each shoulder and draws the blade down diagonally to the lower part of the sternum, also called the xiphoid process. In a female decedent, the cut arcs below the breasts; this will make the "arms" of the "Y" curved. She then slices down the length of the body, past the navel or belly button, and over the abdominal cavity to the pubic bone. This area contains most of the digestive and urinary systems (Autopsy 2005; Timmermans 2006; Gawande 2001).

These incisions will bleed very little—if at all—as a deceased person has no blood pressure. After the Y-incision, the operation picks up speed. The medical examiner pulls the skin back, revealing the rib cage and strap muscles—the flat muscles below the hyoid bone in the neck. The exposed innards glisten with a thin layer of blood. Any fat will have a yellowish gleam. The ME, meanwhile, keeps her eyes open for any abnormalities.

Next, it's time to pull out the power tools. The ME turns on her Stryker saw and cuts through the lateral sides of the ribs to expose the chest cavity, the area between the ribs and the diaphragm. The diaphragm is dome-shaped, made of muscle and connective tissue and separates the abdominal cavity from the thorax. It helps us breathe.

The ME lifts off the ribs and attached breastbone like the top off a box, cutting away with her scalpel the soft tissue attached to the opposite side of the chest plate. These chest bones are often fractured during cardiopulmonary resuscitation. The lungs and heart are now exposed, the latter contained in tissue called the pericardial sac. The ME slices open the pericardial sac to reveal the heart. Very small pieces of soft tissue and blood wash down the gutters running along each side of the dissection table, swirling into the drain (Autopsy 2005).

She slides the scalpel up under the skin of the chest, loosening the skin up to the jawline and then cutting around the tongue and over vessels to release the throat organs. She may now look at the deceased's tongue. A swollen, reddish blue tongue indicates a choking victim. The hyoid, a small U-shaped bone that supports the muscles of the tongue, may be fractured if the decedent has been violently, manually strangled.

Working down the body, the ME cuts the abdominal muscles, pulling them aside to open up the abdomen, or belly. This area between the chest and the hips contains several organs, including the stomach and intestines. She then ties strings to the carotid arteries on each side of the neck as well as the sub clavian arteries. The strings will let the mortician know where to inject embalming fluids once he receives the body (Autopsy 2005). It's now time to remove the organs.

Doctors have their own preferences and may do things their own way, but there are two major approaches to removing organs from the body. In the method named after the celebrated nineteenth-century pathologist Rudolph Virchow, each organ is removed separately and then examined. Some medical examiners find this method the most efficient. In the Rokitansky method, named after another illustrious nineteenth-century pathologist, Karl Rokitansky, all the organs are removed as a single mass and then dissected on the autopsy table. The Rokitansky method helps medical residents learn how to perform an autopsy, as it allows them to observe the relationship of organs to each other once they are removed from the body. A medical examiner using the Rokitansky method may also have a clearer view of stab wounds or the trajectory of a bullet as it passed through the organs, as well as the extent of organ damage.

The first step in the Rokitansky method is to sever the trachea or windpipe, a tubelike portion of the respiratory tract located above the larynx, also known as the voice box. This releases the larynx and esophagus from the pharynx (the throat). The medical examiner then uses the scalpel to free the chest organs from the chest wall, including the heart, lungs, larynx, trachea, and diaphragm. The chest wall is made up of structures outside the lungs that move when a person breathes, including the rib cage, diaphragm, and abdomen. The next step is to cut tissues that hold in abdominal organs, such as the intestines and stomach. At this point, all that's holding in the internal organs are their connections to pelvic ligaments, the bladder and the rectum. When these connections are severed, the internal organs can be lifted out as a single entity for further examination. Sometimes called a "block," this mass of organs is carefully set down on a nearby table. It helps to have an assistant on hand when doing this. The bladder and rectum are usually left behind in the body but will be also examined (Autopsy 2005; Baden 2006). Once the internal organs have been removed and set aside for study and sample-taking, it's time to open up the decedent's skull.

The medical examiner withdraws the body block from under the decedent's back and tucks it under the head. The cranium now elevated, she uses the scalpel to make a cut from behind one ear, over the crown of the head, to the opposite ear. This divides the crown into two flaps of skin that can be pulled away from the skull. The medical examiner peels the front flap down over the face, exposing the top and front of the skull, and then pulls the back flap down to the nape of the neck, exposing the calvaria—the dome of the skull. The ME makes her incision over the back of the head so it can be sewn up later and hidden from mourners who may subsequently view the deceased at an open-casket funeral.

The ME then uses the Stryker saw to cut around the circumference of the skull, with care taken to saw through bone but not brain. She may have plenty of bone tissue to carve through: human skulls range in thickness from one-eighth of an inch to half an inch (Baden 2006). The ME then lifts the top of the skull off the brain as though it were a cap. The outer membrane covering the brain—the dura mater—remains with the skull, or calvaria. With the brain now exposed, the medical examiner looks for brown spots that indicate hemorrhages. She then carefully severs the spinal cord and the tentorium, a fold of dura mater that separates the cerebellum from the cerebrum. The cerebellum is located at the back of the head between the cerebrum and the brain stem. The cerebrum is the rounded structure of the brain that occupies most of the cranial cavity and is divided into two hemispheres.

She lifts the brain gently, as it is soft and easy to deform. If the brain needs to be preserved before examination, the ME suspends it from a string in a jar of tissue preservative (formalin) to "fix" for at least two weeks. If the organ were not suspended in this way, it could flatten. After at least two weeks, the brain is firmer and is easier to slice into small segments for microscopic examination (Autopsy 2005).

Brain examinations have revealed interesting details—including the fact that brain size may not matter regarding intelligence. After Albert Einstein died in 1955, pathologist Dr. Thomas Harvey removed and measured Einstein's brain. It weighed 1,230 grams; the average adult brain weighs about 1,400 grams. Incidentally, Marilyn Monroe's brain weighed 1,440 grams (Noguchi 1962).

Einstein's brain did show other intriguing characteristics, however. Although normally a deep groove divides the parietal cortex in a human brain, Einstein's brain had no such groove. His brain did have a greater density of neurons and increased connectivity in the parietal cortex—this area has recently been associated with mathematical skills (Einstein's 2007).

After the trunk organs are removed, in our example by the Rokitansky method, the ME begins to separate and examine each piece. She will weigh the organs on a grocer's scale to determine if they weigh more or less than the norm—a possible sign of disease. The ME will also take tissue and fluid samples to check for poisons, street drugs, or other potential killers. She begins with the esophagus, then severs the lungs from the heart and trachea and weighs them on a grocer's scale. Normal lung tissue is a pinkish blue-gray color. Dilated airspaces on the ends of the upper lobes indicate emphysema, a lung condition associated with smoking and lung infections. In this disease, an abnormal amount of air accumulates in the alveoli, the tiny air sacs in the lungs. The alveoli become enlarged and may break and form scar tissue as air continues to accumulate in them. Lung scar tissue can also be caused by freebasing heroin. Additives used to "cut," or dilute, the heroin may not dissolve readily and may clog blood vessels leading to the lungs, liver, kidneys, or brain.

Sooty deposits in lungs indicate that the decedent was a heavy smoker. To get a closer look, the ME sections the lungs with a "bread knife," medical examiner jargon for a long, unserrated knife that looks like, but isn't, the type of knife used to cut bread and pastry. The cut segments are approximately one centimeter thick. Organ abnormalities are noted; tissue may be sent for further examination to a lab (Temple 2005).

The ME next considers the heart. An adult heart with no evidence of disease weighs between 300 grams and 500 grams, depending on the weight of its owner. An enlarged, heavy heart can indicate disease: high blood pressure can dramatically increase the size of the heart. Once it is removed and weighed, the ME cuts the heart open with a bread knife or snips it with scissors along the coronary blood pathway to look into the chambers for clots or fatty deposits (Ribowsky and Shachtman 2006). Many hearts show some sign of disease, even when their owners were unaware of it.

The forensic pathologist continues to examine the body's internal organs. She slits open the larynx and trachea longitudinally to examine the interior lumen (the cavity within). The trachea, which connects the nose, mouth, and lungs, will be blocked if the person choked to death, typically with food.

The ME severs the thyroid gland from the trachea with scissors, weighs it on a triple beam scale, cuts it into thin slices, and examines it closely. Located in the throat, the thyroid gland is a key organ in metabolism. It makes hormones to regulate body temperature, heart rate, blood pressure, and the rate at which food is metabolized. A person's heart can beat too fast if she has hyperthyroidism (overactive thyroid) or too slowly if she has hypothyroidism (underactive thyroid). Excessively high thyroid hormone levels in the blood can over stimulate the heart and lead to a heart attack. A too-low heart rate can also lead to heart failure.

The medical examiner then turns over the connected abdominal organs to expose the kidneys. The adrenal glands, located above the kidneys, are cut free, weighed on the triple beam balance, and sectioned. Tumors in the adrenal glands can indicate Cushing's syndrome, marked by easily bruised skin, pink or purple stretch marks, and puffiness in the face.

The ME uses scissors to separate the liver from the remaining organs and then weighs it and sections it with a bread knife. A relatively healthy liver is brown, firm, smooth to the touch, and weighs about 1,500 grams. A diseased liver may be a tan-orange, yellow-orange, or yellow in color and may feel stiff and fatty, and possibly enlarged. A cirrhotic liver—one scarred or permanently damaged by alcohol, viral infections, or other diseases—has a granular texture and can be very fragile. The medical examiner may be able to easily poke her finger through a slice (Timmermans 2006).

The ME frees the spleen and then weighs and sections it. Located to the left of the stomach and below the diaphragm, the spleen stores blood, disintegrates old blood cells, filters foreign substances from the blood, and produces white blood cells. Depending on preference, the medical examiner may use scissors or a bread knife to separate the intestines from their mesentery—the membranous tissue that encircles the small intestine and anchors it to the abdominal wall. The ME slices lengthwise through the intestines, exposing feces and undigested food, and cleans them under running water in the sink. Now she can examine the lumen for signs of disease or anything else of interest, such as wound tracks in a stabbing victim. The ME could also find a tapeworm, although this would be incidental to the forensic aspects of the autopsy. The medical examiner removes the stomach and slashes it open along its greater curvature to reveal its lining. Stomachs can hide surprises. Sometimes drug smugglers known as "body packers" die when the packaged street drugs they've swallowed leak out of their containers. The cause of death is "acute intoxication due to leakage or rupture of packets." She may also see an ulcer or stomach cancer.

The ME must examine the stomach contents carefully, as she may find clues about the last meal and whether the person had eaten anything abnormal. Analyzing stomach contents to determine time of death, however, may be unreliable and could be misleading in court. Digestion is affected by a wide variety of variables, such as the type of food, the amount of food, and the person's health and emotional state. Sudden trauma—either physical or psychological, such as a terrible pain or fright—can be the most disruptive to the digestive process. Food may remain in the stomach for days after a severe injury (Berg and Jaffe 1989; Evans 2008).

The forensic pathologist shifts her attention to the pancreas, tucked behind the stomach. This gland helps digest food and secretes insulin, a hormone that controls blood sugar levels in the body. A shrunken, scarred, and calcified pancreas is a sign of diabetes.

She separates the pancreas from the duodenum—the first portion of the small intestine attached to the stomach—and then weighs, slices, and examines it. The ME then slits open the duodenum lengthwise, rinses it with water, and scrutinizes any findings.

She removes the kidneys separately, weighs and examines them, and then turns to the urinary bladder. Taking care not to spill the urine, she either inserts a pipette into the bladder to remove the fluid or slices it open and ladles out the urine for later analysis. The ME opens up the bladder and inspects its lumen. If the decedent is female, the ME removes the ovaries, cuts them in half, and takes a close look. She opens the uterus and checks for anything relevant, such as signs of pregnancy or disease.

Major blood vessels are also cut open, such as the vessels that connect the heart and the kidney. A coronary artery that is 75 percent clogged with plaque or calcium can qualify as cause of death (Autopsy 2005; Timmermans 2006).

Body fluids and organs are checked for various substances that may show signs of disease or have led to the decedent's death. The ME uses as much of the vitreous humor as she needs to, as it has been replaced with saline solution. She likely will have it tested for digoxin (a drug used to treat heart failure) as well as electrolytes and glucose. Next, she may look for codeine and morphine in the bile. Using a large syringe, she withdraws 15 milliliters of blood from the decedent's leg to analyze for alcohol and carbon monoxide. The ME has the urine checked for most toxicants. She will have one whole lung analyzed for methadone, gases, and inhalants, and a whole kidney for heavy metals. The stomach and intestinal contents are analyzed, as they can reveal toxicants taken orally.

From the liver, the ME takes a sample size of 500 grams for analysis of most toxicants. She prepares about 200 grams of adipose (fat) tissue to check for insecticides such as thiopental. She needs about 500 grams of brain tissue to do a thorough analysis for volatile poisons (Eckert 1997).

Next, the medical examiner uses a sharp bread knife or scalpel to slice one or more sections of organs for microscopic examination, each section approximately the size of a postage stamp in length and width and approximately 3 millimeters thick. Sections are placed in separate plastic cassettes, like tiny versions of the old-format tape cassette containers commonly used in the 1980s. Tissue cassettes are small, expendable containers with hinged, removable, or separate lids. For sample processing purposes, the design allows for the flow of chemicals in and out of the tissue cassette. Some are about 12 millimeters by seven millimeters; others are 13 millimeters by 48 millimeters by 64 millimeters. The tissue cassettes are labeled with the autopsy date and time, the decedent's name, what organ or body part the sample represents, and the signature of the ME.

The medical examiner gives the cassettes to the toxicologist, who gives the ME a written receipt, stores the cassettes in a jar of formalin in a refrigerator, and locks the refrigerator until it's time to analyze the specimens. This procedure provides a chain of evidence for the specimens, enabling the toxicologist to introduce his results into legal procedures that may arise from the case.

When it is time to analyze the specimens, they are placed in a microtome, a machine that removes water from the sections and replaces it with paraffin wax. Microscopic sections are then cut from the paraffin sections, mounted on glass slides, stained, cover-slipped, and pored over microscopically.

Ideally, the medical examiner collects these specimens before the decedent is embalmed, as the embalming process may destroy or dilute poisons present in the body and render their detection impossible. One example is cyanide. Embalming fluid may also contain methyl or ethyl alcohol and may give a false indication the decedent was drinking prior to his or her death (Eckert 1997).

At this point, the medical examiner has finished collecting samples and studying the body on the table before her. It's time to close up. She fits the calvaria cap back on the skull, minus the brain, which will be examined more closely later. She pulls the two flaps of scalp back over the calvaria and sews up the incision with twine, using the same type of stitch used to cover baseballs. If the decedent is to have an open-casket funeral, the pillow under his head will hide the long seam.

Depending on the practice at her particular office, the medical examiner either returns the organs to the open body cavity, often in a plastic bag, or places them in a biohazard bag to be incinerated later. She replaces the chest plate, folds in the skin flaps, and then sews up the "Y" incision with more baseball stitches.

The ME uses a hose and sponge to clean the deceased, places the body into a new body bag, and attaches a nametag to the left big toe. The new body bag is not locked, as the corpse is no longer considered evidence. Finally, she wheels the body on a cadaver cart into the walk-in cooler to await release to a funeral home (Timmermans 2006).

Now she must wait for toxicology reports before she can finish her investigation.

11

---·•·---

EXAMINATION INSTRUMENTS

MEDICAL EXAMINERS USE a broad range of equipment in their investigations, ranging from high-tech computer systems to needles and twine. This chapter will cover a few basics in alphabetical order.

Blackboard/Dry Erase Board: medical examiners record their findings on these boards after removing, examining. and weighing a decedent's organs.

Body Block: a bricklike device made of rubber or plastic, placed under the neck or upper torso of a decedent. The block lifts the chest so it protrudes, causing the arms and neck to fall back. This allows maximum exposure of the trunk of the body before the ME makes his incisions.

Bone Saw: a stainless steel, handheld saw rarely used today because of the Stryker saw; can be used to cut open the skull. Although the medical examiner must exert more effort when he uses the bone saw rather than the Stryker saw, the bone saw creates less harmful aerosol waste (very fine particles of bone suspended in the air). Inhaling this waste or other airborne particles during an autopsy can produce respiratory illness or other disease.

Bread Knife: also referred to as the "long knife," this tool can section (cut) solid organs into small pieces for lab tests, where the microscopic structure, composition, and anatomy of these pieces are studied for indications of pathology. It is called a "bread knife" because it resembles knives used to cut bread, although the blade is unserrated.

Enterotome: these large scissors have a bulb-shaped end for preventing perforation of the intestine when the enterotome is inserted, lengthwise, into the intestine.

Fluoroscope: a device for examining deep structures, including the human body, with X-rays. It has a fluorescent screen covered with crystals of calcium tungstate, a substance used as a radiopaque agent in medical technology. The shadows of X-rays passing through the body show on the screen.

Grocer's Scale: like the scale at a supermarket, this scale weighs large organs, such as the liver. Abnormal organ size and weight can indicate disease.

Hagedorn Needle: also called the sailmaker's needle, this is a curved surgical needle with flat sides. It is used with strong twine to sew up a body with baseball stitches after the autopsy is completed.

Hammer: along with a hook and a skull/cranium chisel, these tools are used to separate the top of the calvarium from the lower skull to expose the brain and its three membranes surrounding the brain and spinal cord. The word "cranium" refers to all the bones of the skull.

Ladle: made from stainless steel, this ladle scoops out stomach contents that may contain food as well as other substances the decedent may have swallowed or was forced to swallow. This could include pills, cleaning fluid, lighter fluid, antifreeze, gasoline, or drain cleaner, among many other products that could be used in a suicide or homicide.

Rib Cutters: these look like pruning shears, the type available at hardware stores, and are an alternative to the Stryker saw. In fact, some medical examiners use pruning shears to cut through the ribs before lifting off the chest plate, as these shears can perform as well as rib cutters.

Scalpel: this long, razor-sharp straight-handled knife is used to access deep body cavities. The ME may use several scalpels to perform the autopsy, depending on how easy it is to cut tissue. Some scalpels have disposable/interchangeable blades.

Scissors: used to snip open hollow organs such as the gallbladder and to trim tissue.

Sink: where organs such as intestines are rinsed under running water to wash away feces and undigested food before inspection.

Stainless Steel Pans: organs are temporarily stored and dissected in these pans. A bullet pulled from a body can also be kept temporarily in a stainless steel pan.

Stryker Saw: also called a vibrating or oscillating saw, this power tool is a small, handheld electric saw used to cut ribs as well as the skull to access the brain. Homer H. Stryker (1894–1980), an American orthopedic surgeon from Athens, Michigan, patented this saw in 1947.

Toothed Forceps: used to grasp and to remove heavy organs from the body.

Triple Beam Balance: weighs small organs, including the adrenal glands (Death 2004; Geberth 1996).

Some medical examiners' offices will have more high-tech equipment than others, depending on their available budget. But much can be learned in a death investigation by using basic equipment.

12

---···---

TOXICOLOGY

MEDICAL EXAMINERS OCCASIONALLY find themselves with people who have accidentally overdosed on some kind of drug—or suicide victims who have willingly
exceeded the recommended dosage. Or perhaps the deceased has clearly consumed a poison, but it's not obvious which one. Toxicology refers to lab tests
for drugs and toxins, often done by a forensic toxicologist at a facility outside
the medical examiner's office. The forensic toxicologist is a scientist whose
knowledge includes chemistry, biology, and extensive expertise in the identification of toxins in people who have died as victims of homicide, suicide, or
accident.

Toxicological testing is time consuming but necessary, and medical
examiners must wait for the results they need to complete their death
investigations. This is often a great source of on-the-job frustration. Toxicological analysis should be performed as soon as possible after a death
because the natural decomposition process may destroy a poison initially
present or may produce compounds with chemical properties similar to
those of commonly encountered poisons. For example, a cadaver's degree of
putrefaction and microbial activity determines a decrease or increase in the
ethyl alcohol and cyanide content of blood (Eckert 1997).

Testing can be a bit like fishing, as the public has access to thousands of
compounds that are lethal when ingested, injected, or inhaled. These compounds include prescription drugs (such as antidepressants), drugs of abuse
(hallucinogens), commercial products (antifreeze and cleaning formulations),
and gases (carbon monoxide). Thus the more the toxicologist knows about the
deceased prior to analyzing his tissue samples or body fluids, the easier it will
be to perform a proper analysis. The toxicologist should know the decedent's
sex, age, weight, occupation, medical history, possible drugs taken, medical
treatment administered prior to death, gross autopsy findings, and the time
interval between onset of symptoms (if any) and death (Eckert 1997).

Relatively common drugs, such as thyroid medication, can be hazardous
if misused. For example, exceeding the prescribed dosage of Synthroid

(levothyroxine)—a thyroid hormone replacement used to control metabolism—can dramatically increase heart rate and therefore the risk of a heart attack, especially if the person has heart disease. A toxicologist considers these factors and others when performing a toxicological screen. When it comes to drugs—either over-the-counter or prescribed—variables such as sex, age, weight, and metabolic rate influence the dosage's effectiveness.

A drug's effective dose is the amount that produces a desired effect in 50 percent of the population. A drug's lethal dose can be fatal to 50 percent of the population. The margin of safety increases when the difference between the effective dose and the lethal dose increases. To complicate matters, some types of food, nonprescription drugs, or prescription drugs can also influence another drug's effectiveness—for better or for worse. In fact, two or more drugs, acting together, may increase the strength of each drug and create a potentially lethal dosage (Drugs 1993).

Likewise, drug tolerance—the body's increasing adaptation to a drug's effects—can potentially put people at greater risk for complications by raising their need for consistently larger doses to achieve a desired effect. This happens because the more of a drug a person ingests, the more efficiently it is broken down by the liver and excreted from the body. Smaller amounts of the drug remain in the bloodstream, and increasingly larger amounts of the drug must be taken to achieve the same effect (Drugs 1993).

A drug overdose is the accidental or deliberate use of too much of a drug with results ranging from lethargy to death. While a minor overdose can cause nausea and vomiting, a person who suffers a major drug overdose may experience kidney failure, coma, and, ultimately, death (Drugs 1993).

A toxicologist's knowledge of how the body rids itself of drugs and toxins helps guide her analysis. Human bodies convert foreign chemicals into structurally different chemicals known as *metabolites* in a process called *biotransformation*. Usually, the biotransformation of a drug or poison creates a metabolite more readily excreted than the parent compound. A metabolite may be physiologically active or inactive and nontoxic, less toxic than, or more toxic than the parent compound. For example, the biotransformation of cocaine produces three metabolites: norcocaine, benzoylecgonine, and methylecgonine. Only the first metabolite, norcocaine, is physiologically active. Sometimes, metabolites are the only evidence of a drug or poison having been in the dead person's body.

The kidneys eliminate most drugs from the body via urine—especially water-soluble drugs and their metabolites. The rate of a drug's excretion depends on the urine's acidity, which is affected by a number of factors, including diet. Antacids (sodium bicarbonate) can alter the acidity of urine and increase the drug excretion rate. Kidney function, however, can be impaired by diabetes and high blood pressure.

Other organs also play a part in drug elimination. After some drugs pass through the liver, they are excreted unchanged into bile that then enters the digestive tract. These drugs then pass into the feces or are reabsorbed into the bloodstream. Other drugs are converted into metabolites that are excreted in the bile. The metabolites may also be excreted in the feces or converted back into the drug and reabsorbed into the bloodstream. Some drugs are excreted in breast milk, saliva, or sweat.

Samples from a variety of body fluids and organs are analyzed because drugs and poisons have different affinities for different parts of the body and are not distributed evenly after ingestion. The toxicologist usually first analyzes organs expected to have the highest drug concentrations. A procedure that identifies one compound may be ineffective in identifying others. When the toxicologist has a limited number of tissue samples to analyze, she uses an approach that will detect the widest number of compounds.

Gastrointestinal contents are analyzed first when a poison was administered orally because residual unabsorbed toxin may be present. Urine may be analyzed next because most poisons are excreted through the kidneys, and high concentrations of toxicants are often present in urine. After drugs or poisons are absorbed from the gastrointestinal tract, they move to the liver before they enter the general systemic circulation, so the liver is tested. If a specific poison is suspected or known to be involved in a death, the toxicologist first analyzes tissues and fluids where that poison is known to concentrate (Eckert 1997).

One way to check for a drug or poison is with a color test, a simple chemical method of identifying a specific compound or a general class of compounds. This test involves administering a reagent to a substance and noting the reagent's change in color. Usually easily and rapidly performed, this type of test is used to screen urine samples.

An example of a color test is the Trinder's test, used to detect salicylates in blood or urine. In this test, a reagent of ferric nitrate and mercuric chloride is mixed with 1 milliliter of blood or urine. If salicylates are present, the solution's color will turn violet. A positive Trinder's test indicates the presence of salicylic acid—a metabolite of aspirin—salicylamide, and methyl salicylate. A false-positive test result, the emergence of a color when no salicylate is present, may be observed in the urine of patients receiving high therapeutic doses of phenothiazine (antipsychotic) drugs (Eckert 1997).

Toxicologists may also use mass spectrometry, an analytical technique used to identify unknown organic and inorganic compounds. This technique has its origins in the work of two scientists: physicist Joseph John Thomson and chemist and physicist Francis William Aston, men associated with the Cavendish Laboratories at Cambridge University. In 1912, Thomson used cathode ray tubes to separate two types of particles, each with a slightly different mass, from a beam of neon ions, proving the existence of isotopes. Isotopes are atoms of the same element that have slightly different atomic masses due to differing numbers of neutrons in the nucleus. Thomson wrote in his 1913 book, *Rays of Positive Electricity and Their Application to Chemical Analyses*, that chemists could use his technique to analyze chemicals.

In 1919, Aston expanded on Thomson's research and built the first "mass spectrograph," the precursor to present-day mass spectrometers. These mass spectrometers use a magnetic field to separate ions according to the ratio of mass and charge and identify a material by its mass spectrum. The mass spectrum is the pattern on a graph of the relative abundance of ions of different atomic or molecular mass within a sample (About Mass 2005; *MacMillan* 1997; What 2001; Young 2000).

Chromatography is another scientific method employed by toxicologists to analyze tissue samples and fluids for drugs and poisons. A term derived from Greek for "color writing," chromatography helps separate, identify, and quantify the chemicals that make up a compound. This method usually does not alter the compound's molecular structure, so chromatography can provide a non-destructive way to obtain a chemical. It can also separate compounds with components so similar that the only way the components differ is in the orientation of their atoms. These components are known as isomers. Digital electronics are the basis of present-day chromatographic systems. Microprocessors, personal computers, and programmable logic controllers can be integrated into these systems.

Mikhail Tswett, a Russian botanist, first described chromatography in 1903. He dissolved the pigments of green leaves in a mixture of petroleum ether and alcohol, poured some of the resulting solution onto powdered chalk packed in a vertical glass tube, allowed the solution to soak into the powdered chalk, and then added more solvent. The colored constituents of the leaves were washed down the tube; the carotins, weakly absorbed by the chalk, moved ahead; and the chlorophylls, strongly absorbed by the chalk, moved ahead more slowly. Soon bands of orange, green, and yellow—each color representing a different substance separated by white areas of clean chalk—formed on the tube. Tswett referred to the bands as a chromatogram, a record produced by chromatography. In thin layer chromatography, a chromatogram is a dried and stained filter paper or plate.

Present-day chromatography also separates colorless substances and bands that are not seen on the column (tube) after these substances are separated (Eckert 1997; *Encyclopedia Americana* 2000; Travers 1994; *Van Nostrand's* 2005; Young 2000). The types of chromatography in use include gas chromatography, thin layer chromatography, and high-pressure liquid chromatography. Modern gas chromatography can detect some substances weighing as little as several billionths of a gram (Houde 1999; Lerner and Lerner 2006; Saferstein 2001; Young 2000).

These toxicological methods are also used to detect potentially poisonous substances—and drugs—in insects at death scenes. Some examples are cocaine, heroin, paracetamol (a painkiller), and amitriptyline (an antidepressant). A specialty arising out of two sciences—forensic entomology and toxicology—entomotoxicology examines insects feeding on human remains at a death scene to determine if the bugs have eaten toxins or drugs present in the person prior to death. This information could help a medical examiner establish the cause of death. This science is particularly useful when the body is so severely decomposed that no blood, urine, or soft tissue remains—or if the body is reduced to its bones. In this case, the insects are regarded as specimens for toxicological analyses in the place of bodily fluids or tissue samples.

In addition, entomotoxicology has been used to detect drugs in cast beetle skins and insect droppings (Gagliano-Candela and Aventaggiato 2001; Introna, Campobasso, and Goff 2001).

Hair samples are easy to collect and store, and human hair can offer telling facts to a toxicologist. Hair grows within follicles, tubelike openings in the epidermis, the outermost layer of skin. It is composed of fibrous proteins called keratins, as are human skin and nails. Hair is formed when cells divide at the base of follicles. The cells are pushed upward from the base, and then harden and develop pigmentation. Hair grows at a rate of approximately half an inch to one inch a month.

One key quality of human hair is that drugs, chemicals, and other substances can accumulate in hair as it's being formed, creating a growing record of drug intake, drug abuse, and toxin exposure. In most people, approximately 90 percent of the hair on the scalp is in a four- to five-year growth stage. The remaining 10 percent of hair is in the two- to three-month resting phase before it falls out. This can give the toxicologist an estimate of when a given substance was in the person's body. Scalp hair may provide information about substances ingested as far back as seven years. If the deceased person has very short hair or is bald, the toxicologist can analyze pubic hair. Methods used to analyze hair include gas chromatography, mass spectrometry, nuclear activation, X-ray fluorescence and emission, and atomic absorption and emission. Numerous drugs and toxins can be detected in hair, including opiates, cocaine, pesticides, anticonvulsants, neuroleptics (antipsychotic drugs), and benzodiazepines (sedatives).

Neither hair nor nails grow after death—but as skin dries it retracts. This can make the body's hair and fingernails appear to have lengthened (Baden 2006; Daniel, Piraccini, and Tosti 2004; *Encyclopedia Americana* 2000; Litin 2003). Only hair being formed in the hair shaft is affected by chemicals or blood chemistry changes in the body.

These toxicological analyses of hair, insects, and other evidence left at a death scene can be highly informative about the cause of death. But not all medical examiner offices have a toxicology section, for budgetary or other reasons. These offices have arrangements with private forensic labs to perform the analyses. One example is Central Valley Toxicology (CVT), a private lab in California that serves police departments and coroner-medical examiner offices throughout the U.S. This lab performs forensic alcohol and drug testing and screens for approximately 300 different drugs.

In 2002, the lab helped police and other forensic specialists solve the homicide of fifty-three-year-old attorney Larry McNabney of Sacramento, California, the owner of a champion show horse. His thirty-five-year-old wife, Elisa McNabney, said her husband had disappeared and joined a cult after they had an argument in September 2001. She liquidated $250,000 of their assets shortly after his disappearance and later moved to Arizona. On February 5 of the following year, migrant workers found Larry McNabney's body in a shallow grave in a San Joaquin County vineyard.

The team that removed the body from the ground included pathologist Dr. Terri Haddix, forensic anthropologist Dr. Roger LaJeunesse, and a criminalist. They noted that McNabney's body was well preserved. They saw no evidence of tissue damage due to freezing and so surmised the body could have been kept in a refrigerator. The corpse was folded and looked compacted. A hemorrhage on the upper back appeared to support the idea that the body had been packed into a small space, such as a refrigerator.

Police found a refrigerator at the Whalen Ranch where the McNabneys kept their horses. Criminalists Jenny Thomas and Bill Hudlow discovered hairs, fibers, and red-brown stains in the refrigerator. A presumptive test indicated that the red-brown stains were blood. Thomas and Hudlow concluded that the six-foot, two-hundred-pound body of the dead man could have been stored in this refrigerator.

Haddix performed an autopsy on McNabney's remains February 7, at the San Joaquin County forensic pathology facility. He found no gunshot wounds, stabbing, blunt trauma, broken bones, or internal injuries—no obvious cause of death.

Police and CVT speculated on what may have caused McNabney's death. Then the lab staff found Xylazine, a horse sedative, in McNabney's body. This drug is not part of a routine tox screen (toxicology test) and may not have been found without the collaboration of investigators. Xylazine is used to control pain in horses and cows and to subdue wild animals. This drug has also been used in suicide attempts and in a double murder in Florida. Xylazine is not approved for human use, so safe levels aren't known. If someone were to take an overdose, this person would feel disoriented within minutes. He would have difficulty breathing and his blood pressure would rise while his heart rate and body temperature decreased. He would slip deeper and deeper into unconsciousness. Circulatory collapse, respiratory depression, and death would follow.

Although it doesn't take much of this drug to kill, McNabney received a generous dose. The lab's toxicological data on February 20 showed McNabney's body had 8 milligrams of Xylazine per liter of blood. That's almost twenty-seven times the fatal amount of Xylazine—0.3 milligrams—that killed a woman in another case. McNabney's liver, meanwhile, soaked up a hefty 69.2 milligrams of Xylazine per kilogram.

The FBI wanted Elisa McNabney, who used aliases and several Social Security numbers, for unlawful flight to avoid prosecution. She was arrested March 18, 2002, in Destin, Florida. There she confessed to an FBI agent that she had poisoned Larry McNabney with a horse tranquilizer—with the help of twenty-one-year-old Sarah Dutra, a secretary from McNabney's law firm. While Elisa McNabney was being held without bail in the Hernando County jail, she used a braided bed sheet to hang herself in an apparent suicide on April 1. Dutra was arrested in California on murder and conspiracy charges and was subsequently sentenced to eleven years in state prison for manslaughter (Bohigian 2004; KCRA 3 2002; Smith 2004; Woman 2002).

The McNabney murder mystery shows how a thorough look at the deceased's lifestyle can help investigators narrow the broad range of possible toxins. The fact that the deceased owned a champion show horse was a clue that helped crack the case.

13

——·•·——

THE AUTOPSY REPORT: NATURAL DEATH, SUICIDE, ACCIDENT, OR MURDER

LIKE DEATH AND taxes, paperwork is inevitable. An autopsy must be followed by an autopsy report. This document is a record of what the medical examiner discovers during the autopsy and is often a source of debate in court. Information about the death and how it is presented in the report must be accurate, readable, and understandable by laypersons, including jurors.

Opposing attorneys may present arguments about many aspects of a person's death—and what's included in the report. If necessary, the medical examiner can elaborate with technical terms in considerable detail during court testimony. An ME must be conscientious about the credibility of the information in the report and the reputation of the medical examiner's office. Words used are chosen very carefully.

This report can be written in several sections (Temple 2005). The first section is *External Description*. The external description of the decedent includes age, race, sex, height, and weight. Congenital malformations, when they exist, are noted. A description of clothing accompanying the body is included—for example, a bloodstained white T-shirt. Distribution of rigor mortis and livor mortis; hair and eye color; presence of dental plates; presence of vomit in the mouth; old injuries and scars; and tattoos and moles are indicated. Fingerprints and identification photographs with the case number are also present.

The next section is *Evidence of Injury*. This is where all injuries are described in detail. If the deceased has been shot, the ME includes a complete account of each gunshot wound: its size in inches (or centimeters) and location in relation to the top of the head, the sole of the foot, or the left or right of the body's midline. A wound site can also be described in relation to landmarks such as a nipple or the navel. The ME will note the type of wound—such as an entrance wound—and how far the gun was from the body when it was fired. Or he may note an abrasion ring, a mark indicating the gun was pressed into the skin before the shooter pulled the trigger. He also notes the location of any damage to clothing and if it corresponds to injuries, as well as the presence of trace evidence such as gunpowder.

To be thorough, the medical examiner reports on the bullet's path as it perforates or penetrates organs, bone, or muscle, and notes details on any exit wounds (in respect to entrance wounds). He will also remark on any recovered bullets and their condition—intact, deformed, or fragmented—whether they are jacketed or made from lead, and most likely the caliber. Each bullet is inscribed with a letter or number, and then stored in envelopes with the following information: victim's name, date, case number, location where the bullet was recovered, the letter or number assigned to it, and the name of the medical examiner who recovered the bullet.

The medical examiner follows a similar reporting process if the deceased was stabbed. For example, he describes the knife as single-edged or double-edged and offers the dimensions of the stab wound, a description of the injury produced by the cutting edge of the knife, and an estimation of the depth of the stab.

The *Internal Examination* section covers the ME's findings regarding the deceased's major organ systems and organ cavities during the autopsy. Any information about the respiratory, gastrointestinal, biliary, and urinary tracts will be included here.

The *Microscopic Examination* section details what was learned from slides with tissue samples from all major organs. These slides may be used in future court presentations. The ME also records the results of toxicological analyses as well as major findings in order of importance.

The *Opinion* section follows. Here the medical examiner uses lay terms to describe the cause and manner of death, taking into account the autopsy, toxicological results, death-scene and police reports, death-scene photographs, and anything else relevant to the case (Baden 2006; DiMaio and DiMaio 2001).

The medical examiner's last step is to sign the death certificate—if the cause of death is deemed unnatural. If the death was natural, the decedent's attending physician signs the certificate. In the U.S., 92 percent of all deaths are natural; 8 percent are accident, suicide, or homicide.

The death certificate is a civil-law document and public record, specific to each state yet based on a national standard for entering information. It shows the immediate cause or causes of death, and any significant causes that contributed to the death and the manner of death. The cause of death is the medical examiner's written opinion, expressed concisely. In the U.S., if the cause of death cannot be established within seventy-two hours, the cause stated on the certificate is written as "deferred" or "pending." In this case, the medical examiner completes a supplemental or replacement certificate as soon as he determines the cause of death.

As public records, death certificates can be highly useful to researchers. The information can be used to identify causes of diseases, leading causes of death, and potential life-years lost to diseases or injury, as well as geographical areas with increased death rates from specific causes of death. However, sometimes medical examiners and coroners are sued because someone disagrees with the cause or manner of death.

It is relatively common for a deceased person's family members to strongly object to suicide as the manner of death. Suicide in particular may be seen as an embarrassment or as something that denigrates the memory of the decedent. Medical examiners and coroners were sued in at least sixteen cases between 1948 and 1995 because suicide was listed on death certificates as the cause or manner of death. The lower court decision favored the medical examiner or coroner in fifteen of the sixteen cases.

Death certificates can be amended for other reasons as well. For example, at the New Mexico Office of the Medical Investigator, death certificates issued by forensic pathologists were amended over a six-year period—and cause or manner of death was amended on approximately 1 percent of these certificates. In these certificates, arteriosclerotic cardiovascular disease and intoxicants were commonly amended causes of death, although the death certificates that listed natural death or suicide were the most frequently amended. The most common reason for these amendments had to do with toxicology (Baden 2006; Croft, Lathrop, and Zumwalt 2006; Hanzlick 1997a; Hanzlick 1997b; Howard 2005; Wecht 2004).

14

---·•·---

AUTOPSY INVESTIGATIONS
IN MASS FATALITIES

IN A DISASTER situation, a medical examiner's focus is usually not on what killed the victim but rather who the victim is. To get to the answer, these medical detectives and other forensic specialists must overcome a mountain of daunting obstacles, such as a lack of infrastructure; the need to coordinate with various agencies and organizations; the struggle to obtain required resources; and often unpleasant work conditions. That's without considering the emotional toll of working on mass fatality incidents. The following cases illustrate how some efforts made in recovering and identifying bodies were nothing short of heroic.

A category five hurricane is characterized by winds faster than 155 miles per hour and storm surge greater than eighteen feet above normal— conditions that can lead to the complete destruction of mobile homes and roof failure on many residences. One of the most powerful storms in U.S. history, the category five Hurricane Katrina, made landfall in southeastern Louisiana on August 29, 2005.

Massive destruction followed. Bordered on the south by the Mississippi River and on the north by Lake Pontchartrain, New Orleans sits mostly below sea level and is usually protected from flooding by dirt levees, concrete floodwalls, and pumping stations. But fierce Katrina overwhelmed the system, damaged levees, and made a 300-foot-gap in one floodwall. The results were disastrous. The hurricane flooded more than 75 percent of New Orleans, the "Big Easy," killing hundreds of people and destroying billions of dollars' worth of property.

Bodies floated in flooded streets alongside rats, cottonmouth snakes, and water moccasins. Dead people sat in wheelchairs. Looting was rampant. Fearing for the safety of their families and homes, some police officers walked off the job. Thousands of people, mostly black and poor, who could not or would not comply with Mayor Ray Nagin's mandatory evacuation order issued two days before Katrina made landfall, sought refuge in the Superdome. There, problems with air conditioning, lighting, food, and assault and other crimes added to the chaos the hurricane caused. One homicide was committed at the Superdome; another occurred at the city's convention center (also a refuge for those who stayed in New Orleans).

Amid all this, the medical examiner's office had plenty to do. But the city morgue in the basement of the Criminal District Court building had flooded, so a makeshift facility was set up in an empty warehouse in St. Gabriel near Baton Rouge. It would stay there for several months. Members of the Disaster Mortuary Operational Response Team (DMORT) arrived to help out. This is essentially a traveling morgue with medical examiners, forensic pathologists, coroners, forensic anthropologists, forensic odontologists, X-ray technicians, and other professionals in related fields. DMORT is a temporary crew of federal employees who take leave of absence from their regular jobs and are compensated for their time by the government. Ten teams were taken to the Gulf Coast after Katrina.

Dr. Louis Cataldie, Louisiana state medical examiner, was charged with the recovery and identification of Katrina's victims. Stored in refrigerated trucks, the bodies were cleaned and decontaminated with a chlorine solution, given identity numbers, and then processed through three forensic stations. At the first station, the bodies were examined, photographed, and X-rayed so forensic specialists could find details that revealed the identities of the dead. Any personal items found with the bodies were inventoried, and fingerprints were taken if the condition of the bodies made it possible. Many people's fingerprints were, of course, not on file, so law enforcement officers looked for latent prints on personal belongings in homes where the dead were found.

As the weeks wore on, the corpses that came in were increasingly decomposed. Some bodies had been left in contaminated floodwaters for weeks, making identification especially difficult. Other bodies bore marks resembling stab wounds—an indication of damage by animals. It was not possible to identify many of these victims by their faces, so the forensic pathologists sought other ways to identify them, such as by scars, tattoos, or surgical implants. People could even be tracked through the serial numbers on their orthopedic devices or pacemakers. Another method of finding out someone's identity was through autopsies. Performed by DMORT members, these operations focused on determining the identity of the dead—not what caused their deaths. Forensic anthropologists assisted this process by interpreting X-rays to determine age of bones, and compiling profiles of the deceased: their age, gender, ancestry, and stature.

The second station focused on teeth—a highly effective way to identify the dead. Here, forensic odontologists used new digital imaging technology to transfer images of teeth into computers for instant viewing and faster comparisons with available dental records. Unfortunately, many dental records were destroyed in the flooding, and dentists and their staff were difficult to locate.

At the third station, DMORT DNA experts took DNA samples from the victims' leg bone marrow to compare with samples taken from families with missing persons. This type of DNA testing—called Kinship DNA analysis—is more complex than the DNA analysis done for criminal investigations, as it is impossible to get an exact match. Instead, the analysts created family pedigrees and worked out the "probability of a relationship" between the victim samples and the family samples. If victims appeared not to have any close relatives, advanced mitochondrial DNA testing was done (Hurricane 2009). Although DNA analysis is a highly accurate way to identify people, it is also costly and time consuming—often months pass before the results are ready.

After all the specialists had done their work, the bodies were returned to their individual compartments in refrigerated trucks. There they waited to be identified, and for family members to decide if they were to be embalmed by DMORT or local morticians. At the height of the recovery, DMORT members performed forensic examinations on ninety-seven storm victims in one day (Hurricane 2009).

The door-to-door search for bodies in Louisiana ended on October 3, 2005, when the death toll reached 972. But the bodies continued to come in, found by emergency workers with cadaver dogs and residents returning to their destroyed homes. Many of these were seniors who tried to escape the rising flood in their top floors or attics. In January 2006, the district attorney in New Orleans intended to impanel a grand jury to investigate if patients at five hospitals and ten nursing homes were euthanized or abused during the days following Katrina (Cataldie 2006). According to the Louisiana Department of Health and Hospitals, Hurricane Katrina killed 1,464 people in Louisiana alone.

Every incident involving massive fatalities brings its own set of challenges for medical examiners. If anything positive can come from these tragedies, it's the scientific and procedural advances developed by forensic specialists with each new experience.

No American catastrophe created more problems and complications for these specialists than the terrorist attacks on the World Trade Center (WTC) on September 11, 2001. That morning, al Qaeda Islamic extremists hijacked four commercial airliners, crashing two of them into the twin towers of the WTC in New York City. An American Airlines Boeing 767 crashed into the North Tower at 8:45 A.M.; a United Airlines Boeing 767 plunged into the South Tower at 9:03 A.M. Both towers collapsed less than two hours later, and 2,751 people died. As a comparison, 2,403 civilians and military personnel died when Japanese aircraft attacked Pearl Harbor on December 7, 1941.

Police, firefighters, and other rescue workers (such as ironworkers, contractors, and engineers) flooded the scene to look for survivors in the sixteen-acre pile of smoking rubble that was once the World Trade Center. Ultimately, more than 91,000 people—many of them volunteers—worked on "the pile" and other WTC-related locations. Yet only six people were rescued alive from the wreckage. At first, rescuers dug carefully with shovels, but it was soon obvious that heavy machinery was needed to move the estimated 4.8 million tons of tower material—immense masses of crumpled steel, iron, and pulverized concrete, with some areas continuing to smolder and burn for months. As time passed, efforts turned from rescuing victims to recovering the dead and investigating the country's largest crime scene (Recovery 2009).

The New York City Office of Chief Medical Examiner (OCME) was responsible for identifying the World Trade Center victim remains—and what a task it was. Although the New York OCME was one of the largest and most advanced in the U.S., it did not have the resources to deal with mass fatality on this scale.

And the challenges were plentiful. After most mass fatality incidents—such as plane crashes—many victims' bodies are found intact and DNA profiling for identification is typically needed on fewer than 500 people. In the aftermath of the World Trade Center attack, however, very few intact bodies were recovered. Instead, recovery workers found about 20,120 bone and tissue fragments. The circumstances were particularly damaging to human remains: the crushing weight—nearly two million tons—of the collapsed towers; fires that burned for more than three months at temperatures of up to 1,000 degrees Centigrade; the water poured over the site to douse the flames; and the time it took to clear the site, allowing bacteria to do their work. Furthermore, recovery workers had no definitive victim list; it was an "open population" (Biesecker et al. 2005).

Refrigerated trailers were brought in to store victim remains until they could be examined, identified, and ultimately returned to their families. But more space was needed. Already on the evening of September 11, New York City Mayor Rudolph Giuliani had reopened the Fresh Kills landfill facility on Staten Island (its name means "freshwater stream" in Dutch), where gray loads of mangled steel, crushed concrete, charred office equipment, and other materials were trucked in from the disaster site (Recovery 2009). There, investigative teams from the New York Police Department (NYPD) and the Federal Bureau of Investigation (FBI) donned Tyvek suits and sifted materials for human remains, personal items, and any evidence from the terrorists.

The landfill site was soon crowded with trailers, sorting tents with conveyor belts, a supply tent, and a café run by the American Red Cross and the Salvation Army. All personal items found first passed the scrutiny of the FBI team before being passed to the property trailer for cleaning, cataloguing, and photography. Forensic anthropologists studied bones to determine if they were human or animal.

As part of the investigation into the attack on the World Trade Center, the NYPD Crime Scene Unit (CSU) documented evidence at the disaster site, designated as Ground Zero, as workers used construction equipment, including backhoes, to move debris that covered seventeen acres and weighed approximately 1.8 million tons. Workers known as "spotters" saw suspected human remains in the debris and signaled to backhoe operators to stop excavating so the suspected remains could be removed.

Part of a side of beef was found in a body bag. Chicken bones, beef ribs, and legs of lamb, most likely from restaurants in and around the WTC, could mistakenly have been assigned case numbers if forensic anthropologist Emily Craig had not been onsite and identified these items as animal rather than human remains.

It was more difficult to discern individual human remains. Searchers found crushed soft tissue, transfer of soft tissue (when remains from one person become attached to the remains of another person), and commingling of other remains. Teams of crime scene investigators with 35 millimeter cameras shot the evidence and remains where they were found, before they were moved to another location, and then photographed them a second time with close-up instant cameras to document them thoroughly. Crime scene investigators looked for any clues to help identify the remains and document them; for example, cameras were used to zoom in on and take pictures of serial numbers found on a piece of hip replacement.

After medical examiner staff assigned a reference number to each recovered item, detectives recorded the number on the border of the instant photograph taken of evidence or remains, and added the number to a log book that included information about the location where an item was found and the date it was found. Debris was examined again and then transported by truck and barge to the landfill on Staten Island, where examiners, on either side of a conveyor belt, examined the debris for personal effects and potential remains. These examiners identified body parts that were coated with pulverized concrete that spotters at Ground Zero had inadvertently missed. Suspected human remains from Ground Zero and the landfill were transported to the New York OCME morgue. Forensic anthropologists determined if the remains were human.

Some of the most damaged fragments were sent to private labs specializing in advanced DNA-retrieval techniques, including Bode Technology Group, Inc. in Springfield, Virginia. Known for extracting genetic material from bones, the company was able to create DNA profiles from 2,000 previously unreadable samples. These profiles were then compared with profiles made for people thought to have died in the disaster. DNA profiles for missing people were made from cells taken from victims' possessions, such as a hairbrush or toothbrush, and a DNA sample, such as a mouth swab, from a relative. NYPD staff obtained these mouth swab samples during interviews with victims' family members at the Family Assistance Center (Conant 2009).

Software to help identify 9/11 victims was made by several companies, including Gene Codes Corp. in Ann Arbor, Michigan. With Gene Codes' software, M-FISys (Mass Fatality Identification System), data analysis that had previously taken up to two weeks could be done in five minutes. The software sorted and compared data from three different types of DNA tests on 20,000 partial human remains and compared this data to DNA data from more than 3,000 cheek swabs of victim next of kin and 8,000 personal effects belonging to victims.

The 9/11 attacks produced the single largest terrorist mass fatality in the history of the U.S. By June 2003, approximately 1,500 victims had been identified. Two hundred ninety-three almost-intact bodies were recovered. The New York OCME intends to keep all unidentified remains until future technology can identify them. Of the 2,751 people who died at the WTC, about 1,126 remain unidentified (Biesecker et al. 2005; Bode 2001; Budim-lija et al. 2003; Bush 2004; Craig 2004; Holland, Cave, Holland, and Bille 2003; Kruse 2003; Leclair et al. 2007; Lee and Tirnady 2003; Simpson and Stehr 2003; Walsh 2004). The September 11 disaster forced the development of new DNA technologies as well as new ways for multiple organizations to work together after mass fatality incidents. These developments can be used by places around the world unfortunate enough to suffer a large-scale catastrophe. The following case shows an early approach to forensics.

On November 13, 1978, Democratic Congressman Leo J. Ryan of San Mateo, California, traveled from San Francisco to Jonestown, Guyana. His destination was the Peoples Temple commune, eight miles from Port Kaituma in the north part of the country. Reverend Jim Jones had established the commune in 1963, promising his followers a life without racism. Ryan brought along twenty people, including fourteen people related to Jonestown residents and members of the San Francisco media.

Earlier, relatives and former residents had told Ryan and the media that Jonestown was a prison where members were beaten if Jones believed they were disloyal to him. They also claimed Jones prevented residents from leaving the commune. Yet some residents escaped, and others attempted to escape. The trip's purpose was to determine if the allegations were true and, if so, to help residents.

Ryan and those traveling with him visited Jonestown on November 17. Initially, Jones and the others treated the visitors cordially by serving them a hot meal and providing live musical entertainment at the pavilion. However, after a few residents indicated to Ryan they wanted to leave with him, the Ryan group realized the welcome had been staged. More residents wanted to leave. The atmosphere changed dramatically. Don Sly, a resident, attacked Ryan with a knife. Although Sly did not injure Ryan, Sly was cut by his own knife after he was subdued by Charles Garry and Mark Lane, Jones's attorneys.

Sixteen defectors returned to the airstrip with the Ryan group to board a twenty-four-seat Guyana Airways Otter and a five-seat Cessna for the return flight to Guyana's capital, Georgetown. But loyal Peoples Temple members followed in a dump truck and on a flat bed trailer pulled by a tractor. They arrived at the airstrip at approximately 4:20 P.M., about half a dozen of them armed with rifled and shotguns. They opened fire on the Ryan group.

Ryan, NBC newsman Don Harris, NBC cameraman Robert Brown, *San Francisco Examiner* photographer Greg Robinson, and Patricia Parks, a Temple member who wanted out, were shot dead. The shooters wounded other members of the Ryan group, including defectors, and headed back to Jonestown. Larry Layton, loyal to Jones and pretending to be a defector, began shooting from within the Cessna with a handgun. One of the Cessna's male passengers struggled with Layton, throwing Layton out of the plane. Although the Otter could not take off due to damage caused by bullets, its pilot radioed Georgetown for help. The five-passenger Cessna, however, got airborne. A member of the Peoples Temple, who later fled through tropical rain forest to a police outpost, reported to police that temple members were going to kill their children with poison.

A doctor and nurses, accompanied by armed guards, forced some residents to drink cyanide-laced punch. Other residents, including some babies and some senior citizens, were injected with the poisoned punch. It was Saturday, November 18. The next morning, the first Guyanese troops, sent by Prime Minister Forbes Burnham, arrived at Jonestown. Jones was found dead of a gunshot wound. A bullet from a .38 revolver had entered his skull above his right ear and exited above his left ear. It was not clear if he committed suicide or if someone else shot him. More than 900 men, women, and children died in the massacre.

The U.S. government took responsibility for removing the bodies because of the magnitude of the human disaster. The U.S. Air Force transported them for temporary storage in refrigerated trucks from Guyana to Dover Air Force Base in Dover, Delaware. Later the bodies were taken to the base mortuary, removed from their aluminum transfer cases, weighed, and placed on gurneys. Teams consisting of one pathologist and two graves registration technicians began examining the corpses on Monday, November 27.

Maggots had infested many bodies. Others were partially skeletonized because of postmortem decomposition. As two members of a team examined a body as well as its personal effects and clothing, a third member recorded results on a chart. Clothing was described, examined for identifying marks, and removed from the victim. Personal effects were described and placed in plastic bags. Injuries and surgical scars were noted as identifying marks. Other information recorded included race, sex, estimated age, and body length. The FBI disaster team took fingerprints from most bodies and took footprints from infants. Each corpse was photographed before dentists examined it and made dental X-rays. After personal effects, believed to be useful for identification, were photographed, the bodies were ready for embalming.

Forensic pathologists from the Armed Forces Institute of Pathology (AFIP) and a civilian consultant autopsied seven bodies on December 15. AFIP is an agency of the U.S. Department of Defense, and specializes in pathology education, research, and consultation. One body had a hard, contact gunshot wound in the left temple. Another had a gunshot wound in the right temple. Brain, liver, kidney, stomach, lung, and other tissue was toxicologically analyzed. Ultraviolet spectrometry, gas chromatography, and gas chromatography/mass spectrometry revealed the following drugs in the autopsied bodies: cyanide, promethazine (Phenergan), chlorpromazine (Thorazine), chloroquine, diphenhydramine (Benadryl), pentobarbital (Nembutal), and salicylates. The autopsied bodies' manner of death was undetermined because it could not be proven whether the victims voluntarily took cyanide or were coerced. There was insufficient evidence to accurately determine if the gunshot victims committed suicide or were murdered.

Seventy-three percent of the 913 corpses examined were identified through fingerprints and dental records. Fingerprints were sufficient to identify 441 of the bodies, dental records were sufficient to identify 73 bodies (Klineman, Butler, and Conn 1980; Knerr 1978; Nugent 1979; Thompson, Manders, and Cowan 1987).

Plane crashes are rare, but inspire terror. Recovery and cleanup afterward can be a colossal undertaking—what's worse, these disasters don't have to be inevitable. The following is a dissection of the forensic investigation of a preventable disaster.

On the afternoon of March 27, 1977, at the airport in Tenerife, Canary Islands, a Pan Am 747 (Clipper 1746) and a KLM 747 (KLM 4805) waited for clearance to take off. Approximately two hours earlier, both planes were diverted to Tenerife from Las Palmas, in the Canary Islands, because a bomb exploded in the Las Palmas airport. It was sunny and clear when the planes landed at Tenerife. The Pan Am flight originated in Los Angeles, California, and had 16 crew members and 378 passengers. The KLM flight was from Amsterdam, and had 14 crew members and 234 passengers. The airport at Tenerife had one runway for landing and taking off with taxiways parallel to the runway.

At approximately 5 P.M., the control tower instructed KLM to taxi onto the runway, proceed to the very end, make a 180-degree turn, and wait for takeoff instructions. As soon as KLM began taxiing down the runway, the tower radioed Pan Am to taxi behind KLM and to turn off at the third taxiway. Pan Am had to be off the runway when KLM would be taking off. There were low-lying clouds; due to fog, visibility was a few hundred yards. The tower could not see the aircraft; the aircraft could not see each other. Pan Am passed the third taxiway and continued to taxi down the runway, searching for the taxiway it had just passed. As the KLM copilot talked to the tower, confirming clearance, the KLM pilot started the takeoff, not waiting for the copilot to finish his conversation. The tower told KLM to stand by for permission to take off; Pan Am told the tower it was taxiing down the runway.

However, KLM heard only part of the radio transmission from the tower because a transmission from Pan Am overrode part of the tower transmission. KLM believed it was cleared for takeoff. As Pan Am tried to turn off the runway, KLM, now aware that a collision was almost imminent, attempted to pull up and fly over Pan Am. KLM's nose and front landing gear cleared Pan Am, but the main landing gear struck Pan Am's fuselage. KLM traveled 500 feet, fell to the runway, slid 1,000 feet, and caught fire. The fire prevented emergency evacuation; all aboard died. Although Pan Am also caught fire, fifty-nine crew members and passengers escaped by jumping through a hole in the wall and through an open door.

Local authorities promptly removed the bodies from the planes and crash sites, eviscerated the bodies, treated them with a preservative, and placed them in wood caskets. This procedure was in accordance with Tenerife law requiring burial within forty-eight hours of death. Many bodies were severely burned or partially incinerated, complicating identification of the dead. The local authorities kept all detached body parts, fragments, and eviscerations. The remains of the deceased Pan Am passengers were sent to the mortuary at Dover Air Force Base, Delaware, where the Armed Forces Institute of Pathology (AFIP), Department of Oral Pathology, provided forensic dentistry support for victim identification.

A dental team consisting of thirty members of the U.S. Air Force, including oral pathologists, oral surgeons, and dental technicians, arrived to help. The team used antemortem dental records and antemortem dental radiographs to identify 199 of 212 victims determined to be Pan Am passengers. Radiographs are images produced on a radiosensitive surface, such as photographic film, by radiation other than visible light—for example, by X-rays passing through an object. Four victims were returned to Holland, where they were identified by Dutch authorities. One hundred ten victims were not identified because they did not have teeth or jaws the dental team needed for their efforts. The Pan Am and KLM airline disaster took more lives than any airline disaster in the world, other than the aircraft involved in 9/11 (Brannon and Morlang 2001; Grayson 1988; Reals and Cowan 1979; Wolcott and Hanson 1980).

DMORT is one of the best things to have come from disaster experiences. These teams are the brainchild of Thomas J. Shepardson, a funeral director and lifelong resident of Syracuse, New York. As most resources in an affected area are not adequate for the magnitude of mass fatality incidents, this network of committed professionals really does come to the rescue.

In the late 1980s, Shepardson, a volunteer with the Department of Health and Human Services Office of Emergency Preparedness, saw much to improve in the ways the nation would respond to major disasters involving mass fatalities. He turned to volunteer teams of professionals in mortuary work and forensic sciences. The National Disaster Medical System (NDMS) accepted Shepardson's plan to create a network of ten DMORT teams, one in each federal region of the country, in 1992. His first assignment was in Oklahoma City, Oklahoma, in 1995, when terrorist Timothy McVeigh used a massive truck bomb to blow up the Murrah Federal Building (Craig 2004; Disaster 2003; National 2003; Thomas J. Shepardson 2005a; Thomas J. Shepardson 2005b).

It's sad but true that mass death incidents have spurred the development of forensic science. Nevertheless, new knowledge ultimately benefits those who are left behind to seek the truth or to identify their lost loved ones.

15

————•◦•————

DEATH REEXAMINED:
WHEN BODIES ARE EXHUMED

IN MOST CULTURES, the dead are considered sacred and thus are not lawfully removed from their graves without good reason. In America, bodies may be exhumed by request of the decedent's family or, under special circumstances, by order of a judge. For example, the family may need to move the body to another cemetery, or there may be doubt about the deceased's cause of death. Other possibilities include incorrect identification of the deceased; the need for further forensic investigation due to an incomplete autopsy; or missed evidence. Often it's about new information that has come to light-whether it's three or thirty years down the road.

While it's perhaps obvious that the length of time a body has been buried affects its decomposition, several other factors are also important. These include the state of the coffin—if it is intact or not—and the moisture content of the earth where the deceased was buried. A body in dry earth may be mummified. Wet soil, however, rots wood coffins and degrades soft tissues, ultimately yielding skeletonized corpses. The clothes may have decayed to the point where they look all the same color—typically black. A cadaver that is exhumed after decades won't contain body fluids, as does a "fresh" corpse. And it's common for a medical examiner to find mold on the body's head, face, and hands (for more information on the human body and decay, see Chapter 2).

When a deceased person has been formally buried and is then exhumed for autopsy, pre-death injuries must be distinguished from any traumatic lesions made during embalming. Otherwise, the medical examiner conducts the autopsy as he would normally. Sometimes stomach contents are identifiable and the ME can have X-rays done to check for bone injuries. He may order toxicological studies and take samples for DNA testing. Diseases such as tuberculosis and syphilis may be detectable in a buried body long after death. The medical examiner will also take care to study the deceased's neck when he suspects foul play or accidental death (Eckert 1997).

Scientific advances—particularly in DNA profiling—have made autopsies on exhumed bodies more productive as a way to solve old mysteries, at least in part. The following example shows a case where both the murder victim and her confessed killer were exhumed for autopsies to solve a mystery—more than thirty-six years after the murder.

Nineteen-year-old Mary Sullivan had been found dead in her home by her two young female roommates on the evening of January 4, 1964, in Boston, Massachusetts. Sullivan was on her bed, her head leaning against her right shoulder with two scarves and a nylon stocking wrapped around her neck. She had been sexually assaulted and strangled. Suffolk County Medical Examiner Michael Luongo attended the scene and noted full rigor mortis and marked dependent lividity. He conducted an autopsy the following day, January 5.

Sullivan's stomach contained several ounces of brownish fluid and mucus that had a slight coffee odor. Her small and large bowels were mostly empty, indicating her death occurred in the morning. Luongo found no edema or external evidence of skull injury, although both breasts had acute traumatic injuries. Police determined Sullivan was murdered by the Boston Strangler, a rapist thought to have killed as many as thirteen women in Boston and its suburbs from June 14, 1962, until January 4, 1964. Mary Sullivan is believed to be the killer's last victim.

Although convicted sex offender and burglar Albert DeSalvo was never a suspect in the serial murders, he confessed to being the Boston Strangler while serving life in prison in 1967 for unrelated rapes. Unfortunately for DeSalvo, although he recanted his confession, in 1973 he was stabbed to death in the Walpole State Penitentiary prison hospital before he could explain himself. No one was convicted of his murder.

Some of DeSalvo's relatives, such as his older brother, Richard DeSalvo, did not believe he was the Boston Strangler. Neither did Diane Sullivan Dodd, a younger sister of Mary Sullivan and conservator of her estate. She and other members of Mary Sullivan's family suggested the killer was a boyfriend or possibly a boyfriend of one of Sullivan's roommates. As for why Albert DeSalvo would claim to be a serial killer, Mary Sullivan's nephew, Casey Sherman, told CNN's Boston Bureau Chief Bill Delaney (January 22, 2002) that DeSalvo signed a book and movie deal to make money to support his family.

As the decades passed and new DNA technology evolved, the two families teamed up to have the case reinvestigated. They consulted James Starrs, a law and forensic sciences professor from George Washington University known for applying new forensic science advances to old mysteries. He helped arrange to have Mary Sullivan and Albert DeSalvo exhumed for new autopsies, Sullivan first from the St. Francis Xavier Cemetery in Hyannis, Massachusetts, on October 13, 2000—nearly four decades after her murder.

Starrs attended Sullivan's exhumation, along with forensic pathologist Michael Baden and several other forensic specialists. At graveside, they noted her remains were almost fully skeletonized with some fragments of adherent tissue. Her body was then taken to the John Lawrence funeral home in Marstons Mills, Massachusetts, to be autopsied a second time.

As DNA technology requires, all those in contact with the remains at the gravesite and during the re-autopsy wore gloves and masks to prevent cross-contamination. Although Dr. Michael Baden, forensic pathologist, author, and TV host (HBO's true-crime show, *HBO: Autopsy*) performed the exhumation autopsy, and would do DeSalvo's too, a large team of forensic professionals joined together to help solve this mystery. These included DNA, hair, and dental experts, forensic radiologists, and forensic anthropologists. Their first step was to confirm that the corpse was in fact Sullivan's body.

During the autopsy, Dr. Baden found the plastic bag containing organs removed during the original autopsy in Sullivan's abdominal region and took samples of these organs for analysis. Although no preservative had been added to the bag, Sullivan's organs were still in good condition because water and bacteria could not reach them. The forensic team thoroughly examined her hair, pubic hair, eyelashes, and fingernails, as well as soil, coffin fragments, and Sullivan's underwear.

A forensic radiologist took X-rays of her bones to look for identifying abnormalities and injuries. One note of interest: Sullivan's hyoid bone (a tiny U-shaped bone resting on the Adam's apple) was undamaged; this bone is often fractured during manual strangulation—especially in an attack as violent as DeSalvo had described. Baden also compared Sullivan's neck and face injuries with what he expected to find from that attack description of DeSalvo's (which included hitting her face and head and biting her), but, as during the first autopsy, he found no bite marks and little bruising to her face and neck.

Genetic testing, meanwhile, focused on mitochondrial DNA (short loops of genetic code inherited through the mother) because of its likely success with aged or degraded samples. Reference samples were taken from Diane Sullivan Dodd and Richard DeSalvo, as they had the same mitochondrial DNA as their siblings. This way investigators could be sure they had the right bodies. A DNA expert also found a substance with identifiable DNA on Sullivan's pubic hair that hadn't been damaged during embalming.

The results of the forensic investigation are intriguing. The tests did not reveal any biological material that could be tied to Albert DeSalvo on the exhumed body of Mary Sullivan. Instead, the DNA expert found mitochondrial DNA from two other unidentified individuals (Foran and Starrs 2004; Kelly 2002; Miletich 2003). Just to confirm the lack of evidence regarding Albert DeSalvo as Sullivan's killer, DeSalvo was exhumed on October 26, 2001, for autopsy and DNA testing—nearly twenty-eight years after his death. The forensic investigation was conducted on October 27.

On December 6, 2001, Starrs held a press conference in Washington, D.C., and told reporters that DNA evidence could not connect DeSalvo with Sullivan's murder. He told reporters that the key finding was that a DNA sample from a substance (possibly semen) found on Mary's pubic area did not match the DNA of Albert DeSalvo. No evidence was found to show Sullivan had been hit, bitten, or strangled by hand. One mysterious detail: molecular biologist David Foran found DNA on Sullivan's underwear—put on after death but before burial—that did not match DeSalvo, Sullivan, or the apparent semen sample found on her body. All these findings indicate that DeSalvo may not be the Boston Strangler (Foran and Starrs 2004; Kelly 2002; Miletich 2003).

Several years before the Sullivan and DeSalvo exhumation, another case captured media attention—and continues to generate controversy today. Prof. James Starrs was also involved with the exhumation and re-autopsy of Frank Olson, Ph.D., a scientist who died under mysterious circumstances while employed by the Central Intelligence Agency (CIA). His exhumation and re-autopsy were requested by his sons more than forty years after his death. Olson died sometime after midnight on November 28, 1953, after he plunged 173 feet to the sidewalk from room 1018A in the Hotel Statler, now the Hotel Pennsylvania, on Seventh Avenue in New York. Olson had gone through a closed window. That's a fact, but how or why it happened is not so clear.

Dr. Dominick DiMaio, who would later become chief medical examiner of New York, wrote the autopsy report about Olson's death. A complete autopsy was not performed, only an external examination. No X-rays were taken. The toxicological report indicated the presence of methyl and ethyl alcohol in Olson's liver. No drug scan was conducted. On the basis of information DiMaio received, he believed, at that time, that Olson's death was a suicide. Many years later, DiMaio would not be as certain as he was in 1953 that suicide was the manner of Olson's death.

On the morning after Olson died, Olson's supervisor, Lt. Col. Vincent Ruwet, met with Olson's eldest son, nine-year-old Eric. Ruwet told him Olson had fallen or jumped to his death. Olson's body was then embalmed and returned to Maryland, where on December 1, 1953, it was buried in Linden Hills Cemetery in Frederick. This was a closed-casket funeral because the family was apparently told by Olson's superiors that the body was disfigured and should not be viewed.

But in 1975, during a congressional inquiry into activities of the CIA, it was revealed that the Olson family did not receive complete information about Frank Olson's death. Nine days before he died, he had a drink with colleagues, unaware his beverage was spiked with LSD (lysergic acid diethylamide, a powerful hallucinogenic drug). He apparently was told about the LSD twenty minutes after finishing the drink. At the time, the CIA was studying LSD to determine if it would be useful during interrogations.

According to CIA testimony, the single dose of LSD in Olson's drink made him behave irrationally to the point that the CIA took him to New York for treatment.

Olson's family also learned that since 1943, he had worked with other scientists to develop biological and other weapons to defend the U.S. during the Cold War. He'd helped establish the Special Operations Division in 1949 at Fort Detrick, the army's bacteriological-warfare research installation near Frederick, Maryland. Olson's responsibilities included developing new secret methods for effective interrogation. During the summer of 1953, he may have been present during terminal experiments or interrogations of former Nazis and Soviet spies in Germany.

The weekend before he died, Olson appeared distraught to his wife, telling her he had decided to resign because he felt his career was in jeopardy. The next day, when he returned home from work, he told her he had withdrawn his resignation due to reassuring comments from colleagues. The secret nature of his work prohibited him from elaborating. He added, however, that he was going to see a psychiatrist because of behavioral problems, including the likelihood of becoming violent. Alice Olson was surprised because she saw nothing in her husband that would suggest violence.

Two days before Thanksgiving 1953, Olson told his wife he had to leave for treatment, believing he would return for Thanksgiving dinner. Olson, accompanied by Ruwet and Robert Lashbrook, a CIA scientist, went to New York, where Olson apparently had several sessions with a medical doctor. Later he telephoned Alice to say he would return home the next day. Instead, he died at the age of forty-three, leaving her and three children behind.

Lashbrook, who had shared a room with Olson, told the New York Police Department he had seen nothing, but was awakened by the sound of breaking glass. Later he told Alice Olson he saw her husband fall through the window.

On July 23, 1975, President Gerald Ford met with the family in the Oval Office and officially apologized to them for the secrecy surrounding the death. Five days later, the family had lunch at CIA Headquarters with William Colby, director of the CIA, who gave them what they were told was the complete file regarding Frank Olson. The government offered the family an out-of-court financial settlement a year later, which they accepted—closing the case.

Yet Olson's family didn't find closure. The CIA's revelations left doubts as to what really happened in that hotel room, particularly for Olson's sons, Eric and Nils. The main question: was it LSD-inspired suicide or homicide? After Alice Olson died in 1994, Olson's sons contacted Prof. Starrs to reinvestigate their father's death.

Starrs assembled a team of forensic specialists and had Olson exhumed the morning of June 2, 1994. Olson's body was taken to the biology department at Hagerstown Junior College. Once the linen used to wrap the body was removed, the forensics team could see that Olson's body was mummified: the chest was flat and the skin was dark and shriveled with no sign of mold. Although Olson's family was told his body was in no shape for an open-casket funeral, Starrs noted that the body was not disfigured. The professor saw no lacerations on Olson's face and neck and no cuts on the front of his lower body or extremities—an odd finding, as Olson should have cut himself on glass shards on the bottom edge of the window as he passed through. One detail of particular interest was a very noticeable hematoma over Olson's left eye, under unbroken skin. This injury was not mentioned in the 1953 autopsy report. Starrs's forensics team pathologist determined that this hematoma was created by a blood vessel hemorrhage, yet no trauma to Olson's skull could account for this injury. Starrs theorized that Olson experienced a blunt force trauma before he fell out of the window.

While Starrs's findings supported Olson's sons' suspicions that their father may have had help going out that window in the Hotel Statler, it seems that's where the investigation ends, at least for now. In 1996, the Manhattan district attorney opened a grand jury homicide investigation into Olson's death, but did not have enough evidence four years later to bring charges.

Meanwhile, Olson's sons continue to believe that their father's death was not a suicide but a murder; that he died possibly because of high-level government concern he would reveal highly classified information regarding a CIA program about interrogations; and that he might divulge information about the use by the U.S. of biological weapons, including anthrax, in the Korean War (Frank 2002; Pain 1997; Starrs 2005; Stover 1999).

One trend in the U.S. could have an impact on the number of possible exhumations in the future: cremation. The cremation rate in the U.S. was already nearly 20 percent in 1993, and is expected to top 30 percent by 2010. One reason for this trend may be the Catholic Church's decision in 1963 to allow cremation. Another possibility is that cremation is less costly, especially as people are becoming broader. One sign of the increasing girth of the populace is the success of the Indiana-based Goliath Casket Company, a maker of extra-large sized caskets. This company's sales have increased annually since the late 1980s. But larger caskets cost more money, as do larger burial plots. Cremation is often the less expensive choice.

The implication for medical examiners and their colleagues is that there may be fewer deaths to reinvestigate when doubt is cast on the original manner of death of a buried decedent. Nevertheless, even though a body may be cremated, there may be forensic evidence at the crematorium—in an urn that contains ashes, or in ashes buried in a cemetery.

For example, it's possible to distinguish resin brands used in composite tool fillings found in burn victims. This was shown by researchers who used scanning electron microscopy (SEM)/energy dispersive X-ray spectroscopy

(EDS) to differentiate the structure and composition of ten modern resins at the Department of Restorative Dentistry, School of Dental Medicine, SUNY at Buffalo. They discovered that the structure of each resin could be linked to a specific manufacturer. They then put resins in extracted teeth and incinerated them under conditions similar to cremation. Using SEM/EDS, the researchers were able to identify the resins after incineration. This means a cremated person's postmortem data can be compared to antemortem data such as dental records to determine a match (Bush, Bush, and Miller 2006; Case 2003; Gill 1996; While 2006).

Of course, forensic experts have much more to work with when they exhume a body than when they work with cremated remains. But a cremated body's ashes and larger remains still have something to tell those who have the tools and knowledge to understand them.

16

---·•·---

CONCLUSION: DEVELOPING TECHNOLOGY
AND THE FUTURE OF AUTOPSY

SOME PEOPLE OBJECT for personal, cultural, or religious reasons to the traditional autopsy with its surgically invasive procedures. Jewish religious tradition, for example, forbids autopsy. But a medical examiner sensitive to religious traditions can take into account a particular tradition and still perform the procedure. First of all, the ME can arrange to have a rabbi present during the autopsy. This ME will know (or will soon learn) that Jewish decedents should be buried within twenty-four hours of death and that any blood, before and after death, must be buried with the body.

One way to accomplish this is to cover the autopsy table with an absorbent material to prevent blood from leaking away from the body or onto the floor. The absorbent material and anything else that may have been used to soak up blood, such as cloth or paper towels, can be buried with the remains. In keeping with the necessary timing, the rabbi can also accompany the body to a funeral home right after the autopsy (Ribowsky and Shachtman 2006).

It's possible, however, that the traditional, invasive autopsy—and the application of scalpels and saws—will become a thing of the past due to advances in technology, namely Multislice Computed Tomography (MSCT). Often referred to as a CAT scan, MSCT is an X-ray imaging technique that allows physicians to observe organs and tissue deep inside the body without making a single cut. Some medical examiners use MSCT as a non-invasive way to examine corpses. This technique is sometimes called a "virtual autopsy." Not only does it not disturb the body—a benefit to those with personal or religious reasons to keep the body whole—but it keeps any forensic evidence intact.

This is how it works: during the examination, a CT X-ray tube and detector spin around the body, taking thousands of images in mere seconds. A computer processes this information into two-dimensional images representing cross-sectional slices of the body. Some MSCT scans provide up to sixteen slices simultaneously with very impressive resolution and detail. A live person may be asked to fast prior to the examination or to hold her breath during portions of the scan to ensure a clear image. This, understandably, is not a concern to forensic pathologists.

Virtual autopsies have also been used to save lives. Since late 2004, the Pentagon has used virtual autopsies to study the remains of military casualties from Iraq and Afghanistan to develop better helmets and body armor. Virtual autopsies were performed on 1,700 bodies received at the Charles C. Carson Center for Mortuary Affairs, which opened in October 2003 at Dover Air Force Base in Delaware.

The only Department of Defense mortuary in the continental U.S., this $30 million, 70,000-square-foot facility replaced a forty-eight-year-old mortuary. Many bodies have passed through this place: since 1955, the remains of more than 60,000 people, including those killed in Viet Nam and the Columbia space shuttle disaster, were prepared at Dover Air Force Base (Comarow 2006; Milhoan 2003; New 2004).

At the Institute of Forensic Medicine, University of Berne, Switzerland, MSCT and MRI (Magnetic Resonance Imaging) have been used to study wounds and other trauma as well as cause of death. The findings were verified by subsequent autopsies.

In a study of forty forensic cases, radiological image data alone could determine 55 percent of the causes of death. Radiology was superior to autopsy in revealing some cases of cranial trauma. At this institute, MSCT and MRI were also used to document and analyze gunshot wounds. Wound channels and bone splinters were documented completely and graphically. Gunshot residue deposited within the skin was visible. Results correlated with the findings of traditional autopsy. This type of scan is particularly effective in locating major ballistic fragments.

In some cases, the qualities of virtual autopsy also offer benefits to the well-being of medical examiners. This type of autopsy minimizes the forensic pathologist's (and any other forensic professionals involved) exposure to airborne agents, such as what may be present during autopsies of bioterrorism victims. Images—rather than slides of contaminated tissues—can be stored on a computer, e-mailed to other individuals, or posted on a Web site.

However, the drawbacks to virtual autopsy are significant—particularly the cost. MRI machines may be priced at more than $1 million; CT scanners at about $500,000. And although these scans are great at revealing bone and metal, organ color (which can indicate inflammation) is not so obvious and different soft tissues can look similar in these images. This type of autopsy cannot determine the type of tumor or infectious agent in a body (G. Becker 2005; Yoo 2004).

Dr. Marcella Fierro, forensic pathologist and former chief medical examiner of Virginia, says virtual autopsy cannot entirely replace the traditional autopsy—although it will be a valuable supplement. "You still need to autopsy to get the bullet," she explained during an interview for this book. "And you won't be able to tell how long the person survived unless you look at the tissue and see the degree of inflammation." She notes, however, that the virtual autopsy is a particularly useful tool for people who study accidents and want an enumeration of every injury.

One thing that will probably not change, regardless of advances in forensic pathology, is best expressed by the Latin expression associated with this medical specialty—"*Mortui Vivis Praecipant*": "Let the dead teach the living."

APPENDIX A: FOR FURTHER INFORMATION

BOOKS

Blanche, Tony, and Brad Schreiber. *Death in Paradise: An Illustrated History of the Los Angeles County Department of Coroner*. Los Angeles: General Publishing Group, 1998.

Buhk, Tobin T., and Stephen D. Cohle. *Skeletons in the Closet: Stories from the County Morgue*. Amherst, NY: Prometheus Books, 2008.

Cohle, Stephen D., and Tobin T. Buhk. *Cause of Death: Forensic Files of a Medical Examiner*. Amherst, NY: Prometheus Books, 2007.

Di Maio, Vincent J.M., and Suzanna E. Dana. *Handbook of Forensic Pathology*. 2nd ed. Boca Raton, FL: CRC/Taylor & Francis, 2007.

Dolinak, David, Evan W. Matshes, and Emma O. Lew. *Forensic Pathology: Principles and Practice*. Boston: Elsevier/Academic Press, 2005.

Dorion, Robert B.J., ed. *Bitemark Evidence*. New York: Marcel Dekker, 2005.

Fineschi, Vittorio, Giorgio Baroldi, and Malcolm D. Silver, eds. *Pathology of the Heart and Sudden Death in Forensic Medicine*. Boca Raton, FL: CRC/Taylor & Francis, 2006.

Hanzlick, Randy, ed. *Cause of Death and the Death Certificate: Important Information for Physicians, Coroners, Medical Examiners, and the Public*. Northfield, IL: College of American Pathologists, 2006.

Karch, Steven B., ed. *Pathology, Toxicogenetics, and Criminalistics of Drug Abuse*. Boca Raton, FL: CRC Press/Taylor & Francis, 2008.

Noguchi, Thomas T., and Joseph DiMona. *Coroner at Large*. New York: Pocket Books, 1985.

Spitz, Werner U., and Daniel J. Spitz, eds.. *Spitz and Fisher's Medicolegal Investigation of Death: Guidelines for the Application of Pathology to Crime Investigation*. 4th ed. Springfield, IL: Charles C. Thomas, 2006.

Thompson, Timothy, and Susan Black. *Forensic Human Identification*. Boca Raton, FL: Taylor & Francis, 2007.

Vanezis, Peter, and Anthony Busuttil, eds. *Suspicious Death Scene Investigation*. London: Arnold, 1996.

Zugibe, Frederick T., and David L. Carroll. *Dissecting Death: Secrets of a Medical Examiner*. New York: Broadway Books, 2005.

JOURNALS

American Journal of Forensic Medicine and Pathology
Forensic Science International
International Journal of Legal Medicine
Journal of Forensic Sciences
Legal Medicine
Medicine, Science, and the Law

DIALOG DATABASES

File	157	BIOSIS Toxicology	1969+
File	155	MEDLINE	1950+
File	156	ToxFile	1964+

ORGANIZATIONS

American Society of Forensic Odontology (ASFO)
13048 N. Research Boulevard, Suite B
Austin, TX 78750
www.asfo.org/contact
director@asfo.org

Armed Forces Institute of Pathology (AFIP)
6825 16th Street NW
Washington, DC 20306−6000
Phone: 202.782.2100
www.afip.org

International Association of Coroners and Medical Examiners (IAC&ME)
1704 Pinto Lane
Las Vegas, NV 89106
Phone: 702.455.3210
Fax: 702.387.0092
www.theiacme.com
mur@co.clark.nv.us

National Association of Medical Examiners (NAME)
430 Pryor Street SW
Atlanta, GA 30312
Phone: 404.730.4781
www.thename.org

Oklahoma State University
Center for Health Sciences
Graduate Program in Forensic Sciences

Forensic Pathology
1111 W. 17th Street
Tulsa, OK 74107—1898
Phone: 918.561.1108
Fax: 918.561.5729
www.healthsciences.okstate.edu/forensic/ms.htm
forensic@okstate.edu

APPENDIX B: FORENSIC PATHOLOGY TRAINING PROGRAMS

————◆◆◆————

Vernard I. Adams, M.D.
Hillsborough County Medical Examiner Department
Tampa, FL 33602
Phone: 813.272.5342
E-mail: adamsv@hillsboroughcounty.org

Andrew M. Baker, M.D.
Hennepin County Medical Examiner's Office
Minneapolis, MN 55415
Phone: 612.215.6300
Fax: 612.215.6330
E-mail: david.eggen@co.hennepin.mn.us

Jeffrey J. Barnard, M.D.
Southwestern Institute of Forensic Sciences
Dallas, TX 75235
Phone: 214.920.5913
E-mail: jbarnard@dallascounty.org

Thomas R. Beaver, M.D.
Lubbock County Medical Examiner's Office
Lubbock, TX 79414
Phone: 806.743.7755
Fax: 806.743.7759
E-mail: John.Omalley@ttuhsc.edu

John D. Butts, M.D.
Office of the Chief Medical Examiner
Chapel Hill, NC 27599
Phone: 919.966.2253
E-mail: jbutts@ocme.unc.edu

Joye M. Carter, M.D.
Indiana University School of Medicine
Indianapolis, IN 46202
Phone: 317.327.4744
Fax: 317.327.4563
E-mail: jcarter@indygov.org

Stephen J. Cina, M.D.
Broward County Medical Examiner's Office
Fort Lauderdale, FL 33312
Phone: 954.327.6513
E-mail: cinasj@pol.net

Tracey S. Corey, M.D.
Office of the Medical Examiner
Louisville, KY 40204
Phone: 502.852.5587
Fax: 502.852.1767

Gregory G. Davis, M.D., M.P.H.
Jefferson County Coroner/Medical Examiner Office
Birmingham, AL 35233
Phone: 205.930.3603
Fax: 205.930.3595
E-mail: gdavis@path.uab.edu

Thomas A. Deering, M.D.
Medical Examiner's Office, State of Tennessee
Nashville, TN 37216
Phone: 615.743.1800
E-mail: irobison@forensicmed.com

Mary H. Dudley, M.D.
Office of the Jackson County Medical Examiner
Kansas City, MO 64108
Phone: 816.881.6600
Fax: 816.404.1345
E-mail: mdudley@jacksongov.org

Joseph A. Felo, D.O.
Cuyahoga County Coroner's Office
Cleveland, OH 44106
Phone: 216.698.5491
Fax: 216.698.6649
E-mail: jfelo@cuyahogacounty.us

David R. Fowler, M.D.
Office of the Chief Medical Examiner—State of Maryland
Baltimore, MD 21201
Phone: 410.333.3225
Fax: 410.333.3063

Randall E. Frost, M.D.
Bexar County Medical Examiner's Office
San Antonio, TX 78229
Phone: 210.335.4053
Fax: 210.335.4052
E-mail: frostmd@bexar.org

Jeffrey J. Grofton, M D
Office of the Chief Medical Examiner
Oklahoma City, OK 73117
Phone: 405.239.7141
E-mail: medicalexaminer@ocmeokc.state.ok.us

Wendy M. Gunther, M.D.
Office of the Chief Medical Examiner
Norfolk, VA 23510
Phone: 757.683.8366
Fax: 757.683.2589
E-mail: wendy.gunther@vdh.virginia.gov

Randy L. Hanzlick, M.D.
Fulton County Medical Examiner's Office
Atlanta, GA 30312
Phone: 404.730.4400
Fax: 404.332.0386
E-mail: mmojonn@emory.edu

Richard C. Harruff, M.D., Ph.D.
King County Medical Examiner's Office
Seattle, WA 98104
Phone: 206.731.3232
Fax: 206.731.8555
E-mail: richard.harruff@kingcounty.gov

Zhongxue Hua, M.D., Ph.D.
Regional Medical Examiner Office
Newark, NJ 07103
Phone: 973.648.7258
Fax: 973.648.3692
E-mail: huaz@njdcj.org

Bruce A. Hyma, M.D.
Miami-Dade Medical Examiner Department
Miami, FL 33136
Phone: 305.545.2425
Fax: 305.545.2412
E-mail: bahyma@miamidade.gov

Donald R. Jason, M.D., J.D.
Wake Forest University
Winston-Salem, NC 27157−1072
Phone: 336.716.2634
E-mail: djason@wfubmc.edu

Jeffrey M. Jentzen, M.D., B.S.
Milwaukee County Medical Examiner's Office
Milwaukee, WI 53233
Phone: 414.223.1216
Fax: 414.223.1237
E-mail: jjentzen@milwcnty.com

Nancy L. Jones, M.D.
Office of the Medical Examiner of Cook County
Chicago, IL 60612
Phone: 312.997.4400
Fax: 312.997.3024

Deborah Kay, M.D.
Office of the Chief Medical Examiner
Richmond, VA 23219
Phone: 604.786.1033
Fax: 604.371.8595
E-mail: deborah.kay@vdh.virginia.gov

Lee Lehman, M.D., Ph.D.
Montgomery County Coroner's Office
Dayton, OH 45402
Phone: 937.225.4156
Fax: 937.496.7916
E-mail: lehmanl@montcnty.org

Cheryl Loewe, M.D.
Wayne County Medical Examiner's Office
Detroit, MI 48207
Phone: 313.833.2543
Fax: 313.833.2534
E-mail: cloewe@co.wayne.mi.us

Craig T. Mallak, J.D., M.D.
Office of the Armed Forces Medical Examiner
Rockville, MD 20850
Phone: 301.319.0145
Fax: 301.319.3544
E-mail: craig.mallak@afip.osd.mil

Henry M. Nields, M.D., Ph.D.
Office of the Chief Medical Examiner
Boston, MA 02118–2518
Phone: 617.267.6767
Fax: 617.267.4931
E-mail: richard.evans@massmail.state.ma.us

Jeffrey S. Nine, M.D.
Office of the Medical Investigator
Albuquerque, NM 87131
Phone: 505.272.8011
Fax: 505.272.0727
E-mail: jnine@salud.unm.edu

Nizam Peerwani, M.D.
Tarrant County Medical Examiner
Fort Worth, TX 76104
Phone: 817.920.5700
Fax: 817.920.5713
E-mail: npeerwani@tarrantcounty.com

Barbara A. Sampson, M.D., Ph.D.
Office of the Chief Medical Examiner
New York, NY 10016
Phone: 212.447.2335
Fax: 212.447.2334
E-mail: sampson@ocme.nyc.gov

Luis A. Sanchez, M.D.
Harris County Medical Examiner Department
Houston, TX 77054
Phone: 713.796.6808
Fax: 713.799.8078
E-mail: luis.sanchez@meo.hctx.net

Lakshmanan Sathyavagiswaran, M.D.
Department of Coroner
Los Angeles, CA 90033
Phone: 323.343.0522
Fax: 323.225.2235
E-mail: lsathyav@coroner.co.la.ca.us

Cynthia A. Schandl, M.D., Ph.D.
Medical University of South Carolina
Charleston, SC 29425
Phone: 843.792.3500
E-mail: schandlc@musc.edu

Abdulrezzak Shakir, M.D.
Allegheny County Medical Examiner's Office
Pittsburgh, PA 15219
Phone: 412.350.4800
E-mail: ashakir@county.allegheny.pa.us

Christina Stanley, M.D.
San Diego County Medical Examiner's Office
San Diego, CA 92123
Phone: 858.694.2899
E-mail: christina.stanley@sdcounty.ca.gov

Jane W. Turner, M.D., Ph.D.
St. Louis University School of Medicine
St. Louis, MO 63104
Phone: 314.977.7841
E-mail: turnerjw@slu.edu

M.S. DEGREE IN FORENSIC SCIENCES: SELECTED COURSES

FRNS   5013   Survey of Forensic Sciences
FRNS   5073   Quality Assurance in Forensic Science
FRNS   5213   Molecular Biology
FRNS   5413   Forensic Pathology and Medicine
FRNS   5613   Criminalistics and Evidence Analysis
FRNS   5282   Methods in Forensic Biology and Forensic Toxicology
FRNS   5523   Forensic Toxicology
FRNS   5533   Drug Toxicity
FRNS   5713   Forensic Psychology
FRNS   6543   Neurochemical Toxicology

University of Toronto
Faculty of Medicine
Residency Training Program in Forensic Pathology
Department of Laboratory Medicine and Pathobiology
Room 110, Banting Institute
100 College Street
Toronto, ON M5G 1L5
Phone: 416.978.7535
Fax: 416.978.7361
pathology.residency@utoronto.ca

THE PROGRAM WAS approved by the Royal College of Physicians and Surgeons of Canada in early 2009.

The twelve-month residency program provides specialized training for anatomic and general pathology graduates. It includes rotations in general forensic pathology, pediatric forensic pathology, casebook and scholarly activity, and an elective.

The forensic pathology residency has three main goals:

- Train residents in evidence-based forensic pathology so they can perform medico-legal autopsies and state expert opinions on cause of death and related issues.
- Train residents about the importance of a multidisciplinary approach to medico-legal death investigation and the role of the forensic pathologist in this type of investigation.
- Train the resident to be an expert witness in legal matters that include criminal trials.

BIBLIOGRAPHY

"About Mass Spectrometry." MDS SCIEX. http://www.mdssciex.com/products/about%
20mass%20spectrometry/default.asp?s=1 (accessed July 13, 2005).

al-Wali, W., C.C. Kibbler, and J.E. McLaughlin. "Bacteriological Evaluation of a
Down-Draught Necropsy Table Ventilation System." *Journal of Clinical Pathology*
46, no. 8 (August 1993): 746–49.

American Academy of Forensic Sciences (AAFS). 2006. http://www.aafs.org/default.asp?
section_id=aafs&page_id=about_us (accessed January 16, 2006).

American College of Physicians Complete Home Medical Guide. 2003. s.v. "Exophthalmos."
"Goiter." "Hyperthyroidism." "Hypothyroidism."

American Medical Association Complete Medical Encyclopedia. 2003. s.v. "Deoxyribonucleic
acid." "DNA fingerprinting." "Hair."

"Anatomic, Clinical, and Forensic Pathology." Microcorre Diagnostic Lab. http://www
.microcorre.com/ (accessed July 12, 2004).

Anglen, Robert. "Taser Shocks Ruled Cause of Death." *Arizona Republic*, Saturday, July
30, 2005. http://www.azcentral.com/arizonarepublic/news/articles/0730tase30.html
(accessed November 7, 2006).

Apfelbaum, J.D., L.W. Shockley, J.W. Wahe, and E.E. Moore. "Entrance and Exit Gunshot Wounds: Incorrect Terms for the Emergency Department?" *Journal of Emergency Medicine* 16, no. 5 (September/October 1998): 741–45.

Aschenbrenner, D.S., and S.J. Venable. *Drug Therapy in Nursing.* 2nd ed. Philadelphia:
Lippincott, 2006.

"Ask Dr. Baden." *HBO: Autopsy.* s.v. "Does a burn caused by steam differ physically
from one caused by a flame?" "Is there an organ that is commonly the last to die?"
"What is the difference between algor mortis, livor mortis, and rigor mortis?"
http://www.hbo.com/autopsy/baden/qa (accessed August 1, 2009).

Audi, Jennifer, Martin Belson, Manish Patel, Joshua Schier, and John Osterloh. "Ricin
Poisoning: A Comprehensive Review." *Journal of the American Medical Association*
294, no. 18 (November 9, 2005): 2342–51.

Autopsy Overview. Indiana University—Purdue University, Indianapolis. http://
www.
iupui.edu/ (accessed November 11, 2005).

Autopsy Procedure: Removing the Organs of the Trunk. Indiana University—
Purdue University, Indianapolis. http://www.iupui.edu/~pathol/autopsy/main/13/
13.htm (accessed July 23, 2009).

"Awareness Training on Cocaine." United States Navy. http://navdweb.spawar.navy.
mil/drugsofabuse/coca/coca_aware.asp (accessed July 15, 2004).

Baden, Michael. *HBO: Autopsy: Ask Dr. Baden,* 2006. http://www.hbo.com/autopsy/
baden/qa_5.html (accessed October 21, 2006).

Baden, Michael, and Marion Roach. *Dead Reckoning: The New Science of Catching Killers*. New York: Simon & Schuster, 2001.

Barillo, D.J., and R. Goode. "Substance Abuse in Victims of Fire." *Journal of Burn Care and Rehabilitation* 17, no. 1 (January/February 1996): 71–76.

Bass, Bill, and Jon Jefferson. *Death's Acre: Inside the Legendary Forensic Lab the Body Farm Where the Dead Do Tell Tales*. New York: G.P. Putnam's Sons, 2003.

Beattie, Robert. *Nightmare in Wichita: The Hunt for the BTK Strangler*. New York: New American Library, 2005.

Becker, Gary J. "Virtues of Virtual Autopsy." *Journal of the American College of Radiology* 2, no. 4 (April 2005): 376–78.

Becker, Ronald F. *Criminal Investigation*. 2nd ed. London: Jones and Bartlett Publishers, 2005.

Berg, Stanton, and Frederick A. Jaffe. "Stomach Contents and the Time of Death: Reexamination of a Persistent Question." *American Journal of Forensic Medicine and Pathology* 10, no. 1 (March 1989): 37–41.

Bernstein, Jeffrey. "Introduction: Drugs of Abuse." In *Medical Toxicology*, edited by Richard C. Dart, 1064–70. 3rd ed. Philadelphia: Lippincott Williams & Wilkins, 2004.

Berry, P.J. "Pathological Findings in SIDS." *Journal of Clinical Pathology* 45, no. 11 (November 1992), Supplement 11–16.

Biesecker, L.G., et al. "DNA Identifications After the 9/11 World Trade Center Attacks." *Science* 310, no. 5751 (November 18, 2005): 1122–23.

Bignall, John. "Baby Smothered by Cat." *Lancet* 345, no. 8950 (March 11, 1995): 644.

Birchmeyer, M.S., and E.K. Mitchell. "Wischnewski Revisited: The Diagnostic Value of Gastric Mucosal Ulcers in Hypothermic Deaths." *American Journal of Forensic Medicine and Pathology* 10, no. 1 (March 1989): 28–30.

Blumenthal, I. "Shaken Baby Syndrome." *Postgraduate Medical Journal* 78 (December 2002): 732–35.

"Bode Technology Group to Identify Victims at World Trade Center: Country's Largest Private Forensic DNA Lab Contracts with New York." 2001. The Bode Technology Group—About Bode/News Releases. http://www.bodetech.com/about/nr100101. html (accessed August 4, 2005).

Bohigian, Sheri. "No Room for Mistakes at Forensic Science Lab." *Business Journal* no. 323201 (February 6, 2004): 12–13.

Bohnert, M., T. Rost, and S. Pollak. "The Degree of Destruction of Human Bodies in Relation to the Duration of the Fire." *Forensic Science International* 95, no. 1 (July 6, 1998): 11–21.

Bower, Tom. *Maxwell: The Outsider*. New York: Viking, 1992.

Brannon, Robert B., and William M. Morlang. "Tenerife Revisited: The Critical Role of Dentistry." *Journal of Forensic Sciences* 46, no. 3 (May 2001): 722–25.

Bresolin, N.L., L.C. Carvalho, E.C. Goes, R. Fernandes, and A.M. Barotto. "Acute Renal Failure Following Massive Attack by Africanized Bee Stings." *Pediatric Nephrology* 17, no. 8 (August 2002): 625–27.

Briscoe, Daren. "Ready, Aim, Fire—Again." *Newsweek* 146, nos. 9/10 (September 5, 2005): 42.

Browne, Noreen P. "Bodies of Evidence: Dr. Michael Baden Uncovers the Truth Behind Unnatural Deaths." *Biography Magazine* 6, no. 8 (August 2002): 74–76 and 94.

Bruno, Anthony. "Up Close and Personal with a Killer." Court TV's Crime Library. http://www.crimelibrary.com/notorious_murders/mass/kuklinski2/1.html (accessed July 14, 2005).

Buchanan, J.F., and C.R. Brown. "'Designer Drugs.' A Problem in Clinical Toxicology." *Medical Toxicology and Adverse Drug Experience* 3, no. 1 (January/December 1988): 1–17.

Budimlija, Zoran M., et al. "World Trade Center Human Identification Project: Experiences with Individual Body Identification Cases." *Croatian Medical Journal* 44, no. 3 (2003): 259–63.

"Burke and Hare, the Bodysnatchers." BBC. http://www.bbc.co.uk/dna/h2g2/A698033 (accessed July 31, 2004).

Bush, Dennis. "NYPD Crime Unit Case Study: Evidence Collection at Ground Zero." PoliceOne.com. http://www.policeone.com/EvidenceCollection/articles/87577/ (accessed August 17, 2004).

Bush, M.A., P.J. Bush, and R.G. Miller. "Detection and Classification of Composite Resins in Incinerated Teeth for Forensic Purposes." *Journal of Forensic Sciences* 51, no. 3 (May 2006): 636–42.

Byard, R.W., and N.H. Bramwell. "Autoerotic Death: A Definition." *American Journal of Forensic Medicine and Pathology* 12, no. 1 (March 1991): 74–76.

Byard, R.W., S.J. Hucker, and R.R. Hazelwood. "A Comparison of Typical Death Scene Features in Cases of Fatal Male and Autoerotic Asphyxia with a Review of the Literature." *Forensic Science International* 48, no. 2 (December 1990): 113–21.

Byard, Roger W., and John D. Gilbert. "Characteristic Features of Deaths Due to Decapitation." *American Journal of Forensic Medicine and Pathology* 25, no. 2 (June 2004): 129–30.

Byard, Roger W., and Henry F. Krous. "Petechial Hemorrhages and Unexpected Infant Death." *Legal Medicine* 1, no. 4 (December 1999): 193–97.

Campobasso, Carlo Pietro, and Francesco Introna. "The Forensic Entomologist in the Context of the Forensic Pathologist's Role." *Forensic Science International* 120, nos. 1/2 (August 15, 2001): 132–39.

"Carbon Monoxide." MSN Encarta. http://encarta.msn.com/encyclopedia_761551907/Carbon_Monoxide.html (accessed August 20, 2004).

Carey, Benedict, Katherine Griffin, Michael Mason, and Rick Weiss. "The Ice Man's Last Hours." *Health* (San Francisco): 7, no. 5 (September 1993): 10.

Carson, H.J., and K. Esslinger. "Carbon Monoxide Poisoning Without Cherry-Red Livor." *American Journal of Forensic Medicine and Pathology* 22, no. 3 (September 22, 2001): 233–35.

"Case for Cremation." *Christian Century* 120, no. 21 (October 18, 2003): 7.

Cataldie, Louis. *Coroner's Journal: Stalking Death in Louisiana.* New York: G.P. Putnam's Sons, 2006.

"Cause and Manner of Death." Harris County Medical Examiner's Office. http://www.co.harris.tx.us/me/Cause.html (accessed July 16, 2004).

Cenziper, Debbie. "Deaths of the Elderly Often Unquestioned." Monday, February 12, 2001. Charlotte.com. http://www.google.ca/search?q=cache:ZYMN70GX92sJ:www.duluthsuperior.com/mld/charlotte/news/s. . . (accessed November 16, 2004).

Cenziper, Debbie. "Medical Examiner Changes Proposed." Sunday, December 30, 2001. Charlotte.com. http://www.google.ca/search?q=cache:Iz3P18ZVcDwJ:www.sunherald.com/mld/charlotte/news/special_. . . (accessed November 16, 2004).

Cenziper, Debbie. "Other States' Investigations Show How N.C. Could Improve." Saturday, February 14, 2004. Charlotte.com. http://www.google.ca/search?q=cache:ZIgJMRzbULgJ:www.myrtlebeachonline.com/mld/charlotte/new. . . (accessed November 16, 2004).

Cenziper, Debbie. "Suspicious Deaths Exposed by Database Reporting." *IRE Journal* 24, no. 6 (November/December 2001): 12–14.

Cenziper, Debbie, Karn Garloch, and Ted Mellnik. "Suspicious Deaths Going Unreported." Monday, February 12, 2001. Charlotte.com. http://www.google.ca/search?q=cache:IP_1SNc4WMYJ:www.sunherald.com/mld/charlotte/news/specia. . . (accessed November 16, 2004).

Chabner, Davi-Ellen. "Pharmacology." In *The Language of Medicine: A Write in Text Explaining Medical Terms,* by Davi-Ellen Chabner, 850–86. 7th ed. Philadelphia: Saunders, 2004.

"Chasing the Dragon." Drugscope. http://www.drugscope.org.uk/druginfo/drugsearch/ds_results.asp?file=%5Cwip%5C11%5C1%5C1%5Cc. . . (accessed August 11, 2004).

"Chasing the Dragon Heroin Use Causes 'Severe Brain Dysfunction, Death.'" Science Blog. http://www.scienceblog.com/community/older/1999/A/199900039.html (accessed July 26, 2004).

Chen, Pauline W. "Dead Enough? The Paradox of Brain Death." *Virginia Quarterly Review* 81, no. 4 (Fall 2005): 130–37.

Christensen, Angi M. "Moral Considerations in Body Donation for Scientific Research: A Unique Look at the University of Tennessee's Anthropological Research Facility." *Bioethics* 20, no. 3 (2006): 136–45.

"Christine Chubbuck." Wikipedia. 2006. http://en.wikipedia.org/wiki/Christine_Chubbuck (accessed December 5, 2006).

Cohen, C.E., A. Giles, and M. Nelson. "Sexual Trauma Associated with Fisting and Recreational Drugs." *Sexually Transmitted Infections* 80, no. 6 (December 2004): 469–70.

Cole, David. "Woman's Death Called 'Suicide by Cop.'" *Milwaukee Journal Sentinel,* Saturday, January 30, 1999.

Comarow, Avery. "Divining Death's Cause." *U.S. News & World Report* 141, no. 9 (September 11, 2006): 70–71.

Conant, Eve. "Nineteen Hijackers Died on 9/11." January 12, 2009. Newsweek.com. http://www.newsweek.com/id/177724 (accessed August 6, 2009).

Covington, Katie B. "A Guide to Swift Recognition of Dangerous Arthropod Bites and Stings." *Journal of the American Academy of Physician Assistants* 16, no. 7 (July 2003): 37–39 and 42–46.

Craig, Emily. "World Trade Center." From *Teasing Secrets from the Dead: My Investigations at America's Most Infamous Crime Scenes.* New York: Crown Publishers, 2004: 241–81.

Croft, Philip R., Sarah L. Lathrop, and Ross E. Zumwalt. "Amended Cause and Manner of Death Certification: A Six-Year Review of the New Mexico Experience." *Journal of Forensic Sciences* 51, no. 3 (May 2006): 651–56.

Cushing's Syndrome and Cushing's Disease. FamilyDoctor.org. http.//familydoctor. org/online/famdocen/home/common/hormone/623.html (accessed July 23, 2009).

Damore, Leo. *Senatorial Privilege: The Chappaquiddick Cover-Up.* Washington, DC: Regnery Gateway, 1988.

Daniel, C. Ralph, III, Bianca Maria Piraccini, and Antonella Tosti. "The Nail and Hair in Forensic Science." *Journal of the American Academy of Dermatology* 50, no. 2 (February 2004): 258–61.

"Death Investigation Summaries." Centers for Disease Control and Prevention. http:// www.cdc.gov/epo/dphsi/mecisp/summaries.htm (accessed November 18, 2005).

Death: The Last Taboo. www.deathonline.net (accessed May 14, 2004).

Decker, Wyatt. "Hypothermia." eMedicine. March 28, 2005. http://www.emedicine. com/emerg/topic279.htm (accessed September 11, 2005).

deRoux, Stephen J. "Suicidal Asphyxiation by Inhalation of Automobile Emission Without Carbon Monoxide Poisoning." *Journal of Forensic Sciences* 51, no. 5 (September 2006): 1158–59.

DiMaio, Vincent J., and Dominick DiMaio. *Forensic Pathology* 2nd ed. Boca Raton, FL: CRC Press, 2001.

Dobuzinksis, Alex. "David Carradine Died of Asphyxiation: Pathologist." Reuters. http://www.reuters.com/article/entertainmentNews/idUSTRE5610CD20090702?feed Type=RSS&feedName=entertainmentNEWS (accessed July 2, 2009).

Donaldson James, Susan. "Auto-Erotic Asphyxia's Deadly Thrill." ABC News. http:// abcnews.go.com/Health/Story?id=7764618 (accessed June 5, 2009).

Drugs, Alcohol, and Tobacco, 7, 1993. s.v. "Designer Drugs." "Dosage." "Inhalants." "Tolerance." "Withdrawal Syndrome."

Eckert, William G., ed. *Introduction to Forensic Sciences.* 2nd ed. Boca Raton, FL: 1997.

Eckert, William G. "The Medicolegal Autopsy." In *Forensic Medicine: A Study in Trauma and Environmental Hazards: Volume II: Physical Trauma,* edited by C.G. Tedeschi, William G. Eckert, and Luke G. Tedeschi, 995–1003. Philadelphia: W.B. Saunders Company, 1977.

"Einstein's Brain." Physorg.com http://www.physorg.com/printnews.php?newsid=2778 (accessed January 15, 2007).

Encyclopedia Americana, 2000. s.v. "AIDS." "Chromatography." "Hair." "Tattoo."

"Environmental, Health, and Safety Articles: Hypothermia." AT&T. 2005. http:// www.att.com/ehs/safety/hypothermia.html (accessed September 11, 2005).

Evans, Colin. *Blood on the Table: The Greatest Cases of New York City's Office of the Chief Medical Examiner.* New York: Berkley Books, 2008.

"Excited Delirium." CBS News 60 Minutes II. December 10, 2003. http://www.cbsnews. com/stories/2003/12/09/60II/main587569.shtml (accessed November 8, 2006).

"Facts about Ricin." *CDC Fact Sheet.* February 5, 2004.

Fain, D.B., and G.M. McCormick. "Vaginal 'Fisting' as a Cause of Death." *American Journal of Forensic Medicine and Pathology* 10, no. 1 (March 1989): 73–75.

Fallon, L. Fleming, Jr. "Carbon Monoxide Poisoning." *Encyclopedia of Nursing and Allied Health.* http://www.findarticles.com/p/articles/mi_gGENH/is_ai_2699003124 (accessed August 21, 2004).

Fatteh, Abdullah. *Handbook of Forensic Pathology.* Philadelphia: J.B. Lippincott Company, 1973.

Fernandez, Humberto. *Heroin.* Center City, MN: Hazelden, 1998.

Ferrant, Ophelie, Frederique Papin, Claire Du Pont, Jr., Benedicte Clin, and Emmanuel Babin. "Injuries Inflicted by a Pet Ferret on a Child: Morphological Aspects and

Comparison with Other Mammalian Pet Bite Marks." *Journal of Forensic and Legal Medicine* 15 (2008): 193–97.

Fierro, Marcella. Telephone Interview by Tia L. Lindstrom, July 23, 2009.

Fleming, L.E., O. Gomez-Marin, D. Zheng, F. Ma, and D. Lee. "National Health Interview Survey Mortality among U.S. Farmers and Pesticide Applicators." *American Journal of Industrial Medicine* 43, no. 2 (February 2003): 227–33.

Foran, David R., and James E. Starrs. "In Search of the Boston Strangler: Genetic Evidence from the Exhumation of Mary Sullivan." *Medicine, Science, and the Law* 44, no. 1 (January 2004): 47–54.

Forks, T.P. "Brown Recluse Spider Bites." *Journal of the American Board of Family Practice* 13, no. 6 (November/December 2000): 415–23.

Frank Olson Legacy Project. 2002. http://www.frankolsonproject.org/Statements/FamilyStatement2002.html (accessed November 26, 2006).

Frankel, Mark. "New Strains of Mad Cow Materialize." *Discover* 26, no. 1 (January 2005): 66.

Fulton, D.R. "Shaken Baby Syndrome." *Critical Care Nursing Quarterly* 23, no. 2 (August 2000): 43–50.

Gagliano-Candela, R., and L. Aventaggiato. "The Detection of Toxic Substances in Entomological Specimens." *International Journal of Legal Medicine* 114, nos. 4/5 (April 2001): 197–203.

Gahlinger, Paul M. "Club Drugs: MDMA, Gamma-Hydroxybutyrate (GHB), Rohypnol, and Ketamine." *American Family Physician* 69, no. 11 (June 1, 2004): 2619–26.

Gale Encyclopedia of Medicine. 2002. s.v. "AIDS." "Creutzfeldt-Jakob disease."

Gawande, Atul. "Final Cut: Medical Arrogance and the Decline of the Autopsy." *New Yorker* 77, no. 4 (March 19, 2001): 94–99.

Geberth, Vernon J. *Practical Homicide Investigation: Tactics, Procedures, and Forensic Techniques*. 3rd ed. Boca Raton, FL: CRC Press, 1996.

Geberth, Vernon J. *Sex-Related Homicide and Death Investigation: Practical and Clinical Perspectives*. Boca Raton, FL: CRC Press, 2003.

Genge, N.E. *The Forensic Casebook: The Science of Crime Scene Investigation*. New York: Ballantine Books, 2002.

George, Diana. "Deadeye Dick: A Medical Examiner Identifies Those Who Don't Want to Be Identified." theStranger.com 10, no. 6 (October 26/November 1, 2000). http://www.thestranger.com/seattle/deadeye-dick/Content?oid=5397 (accessed July 16, 2004).

German, Jeff. *Murder in Sin City: The Death of a Las Vegas Casino Boss*. New York: Avon Books, 2001.

Gill, Richard T. "Whatever Happened to the American Way of Death?" *Public Interest* no. 123 (Spring 1996): 105–17.

Gold, Barry S., Richard C. Dart, and Robert A. Barish. "Bites of Venomous Snakes." *New England Journal of Medicine* 347, no. 5 (August 1, 2002): 347–56.

Golden, Irwin L. "Nicole Brown-Simpson's Autopsy Report." ' Lectric Law Library. June 16, 1994. http://www.lectlaw.com/files/cas45.htm (accessed September 9, 2006).

Golden, Irwin L. "Ron Goldman Autopsy Report." Lectric Law Library. June 17, 1994. http://www.lectlaw.com/files/cas47.htm (accessed September 9, 2006).

"A Good Man, But a Bad Boy." *Newsweek* 99, no. 12 (March 22, 1982): 37.

Gormsen, Harald. "Why Have Some Victims of Death from Cold Undressed?" *Medicine, Science, and the Law* 12, no. 3 (July 1972): 200–02.

Gray-Ray, Phyllis, Christopher Hensley, and Edward Brennan. "Violent Rape and Bite Marks: The Use of Forensic Odontology and Ultraviolet Lighting." *Policing* 20, no. 2 (February 1997): 223–34.

Grayson, David. *Terror in the Skies: The Inside Story of the World's Worst Air Crashes.* Secaucus, NJ: Citadel Press, 1988.

Green, Helen I., and Michael H. Levy. *Drug Misuse . . . Human Abuse.* New York: Marcel Dekker, 1976.

Green, M.A. "Preservation of Evidence." In *Encyclopedia of Forensic Sciences*, Vol. 3, edited by Pekka J. Saukko and Geoffrey C. Knupfer, 1172–77. San Diego: Academic Press, 2000.

"Grissom, White, Chaffee." *Time* 89, no. 5 (February 3, 1967). http://www.time.com/time/covers/0,16641,7601670203,00html (accessed February 13, 2007).

"Guidelines for Medical Examiners, Coroners, and Pathologists: Determining Inhalant Deaths." *National Inhalant Prevention Coalition.* http://www.inhalants.org/final_medical.htm (accessed January 26, 2006).

"Handballing." Dictionary.LaborLawTalk.com. http://encyclopedia.laborlawtalk.com/Handballing (accessed January 11, 2006).

Hanzlick, Randy. "Principles for Including or Excluding 'Mechanisms' of Death When Writing Cause-of-Death Statements." *Archives of Pathology and Laboratory Medicine* (April 1997a): 277–84.

Hanzlick, Randy. "Lawsuits Against Medical Examiners or Coroners Arising from Death Certificates." *American Journal of Forensic Medicine and Pathology* 18, no. 2 (June 1997b): 119–23.

Hanzlick, Randy, Joseph A. Prahlow, Scott Denton, Jeffrey Jentzen, Reade Quniton, Lakshmanan Sathyavagiswaran, and Suzanne Utley. "Selecting Forensic Pathology as a Career: A Survey of the Past with an Eye on the Future." *American Journal of Forensic Medicine and Pathology* 29, no. 2 (June 2008): 114–22.

Hardy, D.L. "Fatal Rattlesnake Envenomation in Arizona: 1969–1984." *Journal of Toxicology and Clinical Toxicology* 24, no. 1 (1986): 1–10.

Haskell, Neal H., Wayne D. Lord, and Jason H. Byrd. "Collection of Entomological Evidence During Death Investigations." In *Forensic Entomology: The Utility of Arthropods in Legal Investigations*, edited by Jason H. Byrd and James L. Castner, 81–120. Boca Raton, FL: CRC Press, 2001.

Hassanian-Moghaddam, Hossein, and Zahra Abolmasoumi. "Consequence of Body Packing of Illicit Drugs." http://razi.ams.ac.ir/AIM/07101/006.htm (accessed July 7, 2009).

Havill, Adrian. *While Innocents Slept: A Story of Revenge, Murder, and SIDS.* New York: St. Martin's Press, 2001.

Hayes, W.J., Jr. "Mortality in 1969 from Pesticides, Including Aerosols." *Archives of Environmental Health* 31, no. 2 (March/April 1976): 61–72.

Hellier, Catherine, and Robert Connolly. "Cause of Death in Judicial Hanging: A Review and Case Study." *Medicine, Science, and the Law* 49, no. 1 (January 2009): 18–26.

Hellmich, Nanci. "Son's Suicide Prodded Collins to Write," Monday, June 18, 2007. USATODAY.com. http://usatoday.com/ (accessed July 23, 2009).

Henkel, John. "Curbing the Staggering Suicide Rate." *FDA Consumer* 39, no. 1 (January/ February 2005): 39.

"Hi-Fi Murders." Wikipedia. http://en.wikipedia.org/wiki/Hi-Fi_Murders (accessed October 22, 2006).

Hill, Michael D., Perry W. Cooper, and James R. Perry. "Chasing the Dragon—Neurological Toxicity Associated with Inhalation of Heroin Vapour: Case Report." *Canadian Medical Association Journal* 162, no. 2 (January 25, 2000): 236–38.

Hirvonen, J. "Some Aspects on Death in the Cold and Concomitant Frostbites." *International Journal of Circumpolar Health* 59, no. 2 (April 2000): 131–36.

Hochmeister, M.N., M. Whelan, U.V. Borer, C. Gehrig, S. Binda, A Berzianovich, E. Rauch, and R. Dirnhofer. "Effects of Toluidine Blue and Destaining Reagents Used in Sexual Assault Examinations on the Ability to Obtain DNA Profiles from Postcoital Vaginal Swabs." *Journal of Forensic Sciences* 42, no. 2 (March 1997): 316–19.

Holland, M.M., C.A. Cave, C.A. Holland, and T.W. Bille. "Development of a Quality, High Throughput DNA Analysis Procedure for Skeletal Samples to Assist with the Identification of Victims from the World Trade Center Attacks." *Croatian Medical Journal* 44, no. 3 (June 2003): 264–72.

Houde, John. *Crime Lab: A Guide for Nonscientists.* Ventura, CA: Calico Press, 1999.

"How Stingrays Kill." Spero News, September 4, 2006. http://www.speroforum.com/ site/article.asp?id (accessed September 9, 2006).

Howard, John D. "General Principles, Practices, and Guidelines for Death Investigation by the Pierce County Medical Examiner's Office." Pierce County Medical Examiner. http://www.co.pierce.wa.us/pc/abtus/ourorg/me/guide.htm (accessed July 13, 2009).

Howard, John D. "Pierce County: Medical Examiner." September 13, 2005. http:// www.co.pierce.wa.us/text/abtus/ourorg/me/guide.htm (accessed November 18, 2005).

"Hurricane Katrina." Louisiana Department of Health and Hospitals. 2009. http:// www.dhh.louisiana.gov/offices/?ID=192 (accessed August 5, 2009).

"Hypothermia." MayoClinic.com. June 10, 2005. http://www.mayoclinic.com/invoke.cfm?id=DS00333 (accessed September 11, 2005).

Ilano, Aaron L., and Thomas A. Raffin. "Management of Carbon Monoxide Poisoning." Chest. http://www.findarticles.com/p/articles/mi_m0984/is n1_v97/ai_13309787 (accessed August 21, 2004).

Introna, Francesco, Carlo Pietro Campobasso, and Madison Lee Goff. "Entomotoxicology." *Forensic Science International* 120, nos. 1/2 (August 15, 2001): 42–47.

Jeha, Lara, and Cathy A. Sila. "Neurological Complications of West Nile Virus." The Cleveland Clinic Disease Management Project, January 23, 2004. http://www. clevelandclinicmeded.com/diseasemanagement/neurology/wnv_neuro/wnv_neuro.htm (accessed October 2, 2006).

Jones, C. "Suspicious Death Related to Gamma-Hydroxybutyrate (GHB) Toxicity." *Journal of Clinical Forensic Medicine* 8, no. 2 (June 2001): 74–76.

Jonnes, Jill. *Hep-Cats, Narcs, and Pipe Dreams: A History of America's Romance with Illegal Drugs.* New York: Scribner, 1996.

Kales, Stephen N. "Carbon Monoxide Intoxication." American Family Physician. http://www.findarticles.com/p/articles/mi_m3225/is_n6_v48/ai_14658183 (accessed August 21, 2004).

Kappel, Kenneth R. *Chappaquiddick Revealed: What Really Happened.* New York: Shapolsky Publishers, 1989.

Kaye, Brian H. *Science and the Detective: Selected Reading in Forensic Science.* New York: Weinheim, 1995.

KCRA 3 Television Homepage News. http://www.kcra.com/news/ (accessed November 18, 2006).

Kearney, Michael S., Lauritz B. Dahl, and Helge Stalsberg. "Can a Cat Smother and Kill a Baby?" *British Medical Journal* 285, no. 6344 (September 18, 1982): 777.

Kelly, Susan. *The Boston Stranglers.* New York: Pinnacle Books, 2002.

Kenworthy, Tom. "Life, Death and a Load of Loot in Las Vegas: Casino Operator Leaves $3.5 Million Stash of Silver—and a Few Questions." *The Washington Post,* Final Edition, Thursday, October 1, 1998, Page A1.

Keppel, Robert D., and William J. Birnes. *Signature Killers.* New York: Pocket Books, 1997.

"Kim Probably Died 2 Days Before He Was Found." kgw.com http://www.kgw.com/news-local/stories/kgw_120506_news_missing_family_tues.56940 . . . (accessed December 31, 2006).

King, Gary C. *An Early Grave.* New York: St. Martin's Paperbacks, 2001.

"King County Medical Examiner's Office: Policies and Procedures: Chapter 5: Law Enforcement Agencies and the Medical Examiner." Public Health Seattle and King County. http://www.metrokc.gov/health/examiner/policy/law.htm (accessed November 29, 2005).

Klineman, George, Sherman Butler, and David Conn. *The Cult That Died: The Tragedy of Jim Jones and the Peoples Temple.* New York: G.P. Putnam's Sons, 1980.

Knerr, M.E. *Suicide in Guyana.* New York: Belmont Tower Books, 1978.

Knight, Bernard. "Ricin: A Potent Homicidal Poison." *British Medical Journal* 1, no. 6159 (February 3, 1979): 350–51.

Knight, Bernard. *Simpson's Forensic Medicine.* 11th ed. London: Arnold, 1997.

Knight, Bernard, Andrew Barclay, and Roger Mann. "Suicide by Injection of Snake Venom." *Forensic Science* 10, no. 2 (September/October 1977): 141–45.

Koehler, Steven A., and Cyril H. Wecht. *Postmortem: Establishing the Cause of Death.* Buffalo: Firefly Books, 2006.

Kolecki, P. "Delayed Toxic Reaction Following Massive Bee Envenomation." *Annals of Emergency Medicine* 33, no. 1 (January 1999): 114–16.

Kornblum, R.N. "Effects of the Taser in Fatalities Involving Police Confrontation." *Journal of Forensic Sciences* 36, no. 2 (March 1991): 434–38.

Kruse, Melissa. "Soul Searching." Bio-IT World, September 11, 2003. http://www.bio-itworld.com/archive/091103/soul.html (accessed January 19, 2005).

Langley, R., and D. Sumner. "Pesticide Mortality in the United States 1979–1988." *Veterinary and Human Toxicology* 44, no. 2 (April 2002): 101–05.

Langlois, N.E.I., and G.A. Gresham. "The Ageing of Bruises: A Review and Study of the Color Changes with Time." *Forensic Science International* 50 (1991): 227–38.

Lardner, James, and Thomas Reppetto. *NYPD: A City and Its Police.* New York: Henry Holt and Company, 2000.

Leclair, Benoit, et al. "Bioinformatics and Human Identification in Mass Fatality Incidents: The World Trade Center Disaster." *Journal of Forensic Sciences* 52, no. 4 (July 2007): 806–19.

Lee, Henry C., and Frank Tirnady. *Blood Evidence: How DNA Is Revolutionizing the Way We Solve Crimes.* Cambridge, MA: Perseus, 2003.

Lerner, K. Lee, and Brenda Wilmoth Lerner, eds. *World of Forensic Science.* Detroit: Thomson/Gale, 2006.

Libiseller, Kathrin, Marion Pavlic, Petra Grubwieser, and Walter Rabl. "Ecstasy—Deadly Risk Even Outside Rave Parties." *Forensic Science International* 153, nos. 2/3 (October 29, 2005): 227–30.

Litin, Scott C., editor-in-chief. *Mayo Clinic Family Health Book.* 3rd ed. New York: HarperResource, 2003.

Long, Steven. *Out of Control.* New York: St. Martin's Paperbacks, 2004.

Lundstrom, M., and R. Sharpe. "Getting Away with Murder." *Public Welfare* 49, no. 3 (Summer 1991): 18–29.

Lynton, Richard C., and Timothy E. Albertson. "Amphetamines and Designer Drugs." In *Medical Toxicology,* edited by Richard C. Dart, 1071–83. 3rd ed. Philadelphia: Lippincott Williams & Wilkins, 2004.

MacGowan, Douglas. "William Burke and William Hare." Crime Library. www.crime-library.com/serial9/burke-hare (accessed August 1, 2004).

MacMillan Encyclopedia of Chemistry. 1997. s.v. "Cyanide and the Nitrile Functional Group." "Mass Spectrometry."

Macy, Robert. "Deputy Says 24 Tons of Silver Removed From Vault." Associated Press State and Local Wire, Monday, August 23, 1999.

Maddy, K.T., S. Edmiston, and D. Richmond. "Illness, Injuries, and Deaths from Pesticide Exposures in California 1949–1988." *Reviews of Environmental Contamination and Toxicology* 114 (1990): 57–123.

"Man, 79, Charged in Cleaver Attack on Wife." RedOrbit—Oddities. August 23, 2005. http://www.redorbit.com/news/display?id=217710&source=r_oddities (accessed September 13, 2006).

Mann, Robert, and Miryam Ehrlich Williamson. *Forensic Detective: How I Cracked the World's Toughest Cases.* New York: Ballantine Books, 2006.

"The Marilyn Tapes." CBS News 48 Hours Mystery. August 1, 2006. http://www.cbsnews.com/stories/2006/04/20/48hours/main1524970.shtml (accessed December 14, 2006).

Marlowe, Ann. *How to Stop Time: Heroin from A to Z.* New York: Basic Books, 1999.

Marraccini, J.V., G.E. Thomas, J.P. Ongley, C.D. Pfaffenberger, J.H. Davis, and L.R. Bednarczyk. "Death and Injury Caused by Methyl Bromide, an Insecticide Fumigant." *Journal of Forensic Sciences* 28, no. 3 (July 1983): 601–07.

Martin, W.D., J.W. Nemitz, A. Hendley, R.M. Fisk, and J.P. Wells. "Three Years of Experience with a Dissection Table Ventilation System." *Clinical Anatomy* (New York) 8, no. 4 (1995): 297–302.

Mathers, Lawrence H., and Lorry R. Frankel. "Brain Death." In *Nelson Textbook of Pediatrics.* 18th ed., edited by Robert M. Kliegman. Philadelphia: Saunders, 2007.

McKenna, W.R. "The Africanized Honey Bee." *Allergy Proceedings* 13, no. 1 (January/February 1992): 7–10.

"Mechanic Acquitted in Gerulaitis Death." WCBS 88 News Radio. http://ny.yahoo.com/external/wcbs_radio/stories/8444607590.html (accessed August 22, 2004).

"Men May Be More Susceptible to Head Injury Than Women, Study Suggests." Science Daily. January 22, 2008. http://www.sciencedaily.com/releases/2008/01/080121122138.htm (accessed July 23, 2009).

Merigian, K.S., and K. Blaho. "Envenomation from the Brown Recluse Spider: Review of Mechanism and Treatment Options." *American Journal of Therapeutics* 3, no. 10 (October 1996): 724–34.

Miletich, John J. *Homicide Investigation: An Introduction.* Lanham, MD: Scarecrow Press, 2003.

Milhoan, Cathy. "Final Journey." *Citizen Airman* 55, no. 3 (June 2003): 10–11.

Mizukami, Hajime, Keiko Shimizu, Hiroshi Shiono, Takashi Uezono, and Masahiro Sasaki. "Forensic Diagnosis of Death from Cold." *Legal Medicine* 1, no. 4 (December 1999): 204–09.

Morgan, D.L., H.W. Blair, and R.P. Ramsey. "Suicide Attempt by the Intravenous Injection of Rattlesnake Venom." *Southern Medical Journal* 99, no. 3 (March 2006): 282–84.

Mori, Kenjiro, Koh Shingu, and Shinichi Nakao. "Brain Death." In *Miller's Anesthesia*, edited by Ronald D. Miller. 7th ed. Philadelphia: Churchill Livingstone/Elsevier, 2009.

Morris, David. "State Treasurer Had Learned Day Before Suicide of Pardon Denial." *The Associated Press* (January, 1987).

Murphy, John. "How the Eye Is Used in Forensic Medicine, and How You Can Help Detect and Prevent Crimes." November 15, 2004. Review of Optometry Online. http://www.revoptom.com/index.asp?page=21266.htm (accessed July 23, 2009).

Nakagawa, Thomas A., and Edward E. Conway, Jr. "Shaken Baby Syndrome: Recognizing and Responding to a Lethal Danger." *Contemporary Pediatrics* 21, no. 3 (March 2004): 37–39, 43–44, and 47–48.

National Association of Medical Examiners (NAME). June 12, 2004. http://thename.org/ (accessed November 1, 2006).

National Association of Medical Examiners (NAME). *Preliminary Report on America's Medicolegal Offices*. Atlanta: National Association of Medical Examiners, n.d.

New Encyclopaedia Britannica. 2005. s.v. "Bovine spongiform encephalopathy." "Hair." "Prion."

"New Mortuary Facility Opens at Dover." *Army Logistician* 36, no. 1 (January/February 2004): 50.

Newton, Michael. *Rope: The Twisted Life and Crimes of Harvey Glatman*. New York: Pocket Books, 1998.

Nicholson, Katherine L., and Robert L. Balster. "GHB: A New and Novel Drug of Abuse." *Drug and Alcohol Dependence* 63, no. 1 (June 1, 2001): 1–22.

Noguchi, T. "Photo and Excerpt of Marilyn Monroe Autopsy." August 13, 1962. http://www.deadmart.com/monroe.html (accessed November 29, 2003).

Noguchi, Thomas T., and Joseph Di Mona. *Coroner*. New York: Pocket Books, 1983.

Nolte, Kurt B., David G. Taylor, and Jonathan Y. Richmond. "Biosafety Considerations for Autopsy." *American Journal of Forensic Medicine and Pathology* 23, no. 2 (April 2002): 107–22.

Nugent, John Peer. *White Night*. New York: Rawson, Wade Publishers, 1979.

Nunnelee, J.D. "Brown Recluse Spider Bites: A Case Report." *Journal of Perianesthetic Nursing* 21, no. 1 (February 2006): 12–15.

O'Connell, Peter. "Binion Jury Sees Full Magnitude of Silver Fortune." *Las Vegas Review Journal*, Final Edition, Saturday, April 29, 2000, Page 1A.

Owen, David. *Hidden Evidence: 40 True Crimes and How Forensic Science Helped Solve Them*. Buffalo: Firefly Books, 2000.

Pain, Stephanie. "Who Killed Frank Olson?" *New Scientist* 154, no. 2081 (May 10, 1997).

Palmeri, A., S. Pichini, R. Pacifici, P. Zuccaro, and A. Lopez. "Drugs in Nails: Physiology, Pharmacokinetics, and Forensic Toxicology." *Clinical Pharmacokinetics* 38, no. 2 (February 2000): 95–110.

Parent, Richard. "Deaths During Police Intervention." *FBI Law Enforcement Bulletin* 75, no. 4 (April 2006): 18–22.

"Pennsylvania Official Kills Self at News Conference." The San Diego Union-Tribune (January/1987): A12.

"Pennsylvania Official's Suicide May Be Linked to Finances." The Washington Post (January, 1987): A9.

"Perforated Septum." Genesis Health System. http://www.genesishealth.com/micromedex/detaileddisease/00060270.aspx?style=po (accessed July 11, 2004).

Petersen, Lyle R., and Anthony A. Marfin. "West Nile Virus: A Primer for the Clinician." *Annals of Internal Medicine* 137, no. 3 (August 6, 2002): 173–79.

"Picture of Septal Perforation." *Otolaryngology Houston.* http://www.ghorayeb.com/SeptalPerforation.html (accessed July 15, 2004).

Pollak, S., and P.J. Saukko. "Defense Wounds." In *Encyclopedia of Forensic Sciences,* Vol. 1, edited by Pekka J. Saukko and Geoffrey C. Knupfer, 374–78. San Diego: Academic Press, 2000.

Pounder, D.J. "Autopsy." In *Encyclopedia of Forensic Sciences,* Vol. 3, edited by Pekka J. Saukko and Geoffrey C. Knupfer, 1155–61. San Diego: Academic Press, 2000.

Pounder, Derrick J. "Bodies from Water." *University of Dundee Department of Forensic Medicine Lecture Notes,"* 1992.

Prusiner, Stanley B. "Prions." *Scientific American* 251, no. 10 (October 1984): 50–59.

Puswella, Amal, Mike DeVita, and Robert M. Arnold. "Declaring Brain Death: The Neurological Criteria." *Journal of Palliative Medicine* 8, no. 3 (2005): 640–41.

Quatrehomme, G., and M.Y. Iscan. "Gunshot Wounds to the Skull: Comparison of Entries and Exits." *Forensic Science International* 94, nos. 1/2 (June 1998): 141–46.

Ramsland, Katherine. *The Forensic Science of C.S.I.* New York: Berkley Boulevard Books, 2001.

Ramsland, Katherine. "Richard Kuklinski: The Iceman." Court TV's Crime Library. http://www.crimelibrary.com/notorious_murders/mass/kuklinski/index_1.html?sect=8 (accessed July 15, 2005).

Reals, W.J., and W.R. Cowan. "Forensic Pathology and Mass Casualties." *Human Pathology* 10, no. 2 (March 1979): 133–36.

Reay, D.T., and J.W. Eisele. "Sexual Abuse and Death of an Elderly Lady by 'Fisting.'" *American Journal of Forensic Medicine and Pathology* 4, no. 4 (December 1983): 347–49.

Reay, Donald T. "Suspect Restraint and Sudden Death." *FBI Law Enforcement Bulletin* 65, no. 5 (May 1996): 22–25.

"Recovery." New York State Museum. 2009. http://www.nysm.gov/wtc/recovery/index/html (accessed August 6, 2009).

R4: Histology Cassettes, Base Moulds, Biopsy Foam Pads, and Cassette Storage. ProSciTech. http://www.proscitech.com.au/cataloguex/online.asp?page=R4 (accessed July 24, 2009).

Ribowsky, Shiya, and Tom Shachtman. *Dead Center: Behind the Scenes at the World's Largest Medical Examiner's Office.* New York: Regan, 2006.

Rivera, Ray. "Asphyxia, Cocaine Cited in Death at Sea-Tac Airport." seattletimes.com, Tuesday, December 2, 2003. http://seattletimes.nwsource.com/html/localnews/2001805219_seatacdeath02m.html (accessed July 11, 2004).

Robinson, Richard, editor-in-chief. *Biology.* Volumes 1–4. New York: Macmillan Reference U.S.A., 2002.

Ropp, Kevin L. "Sudafed Tamperer Gets Life Sentence." *FDA Consumer* 27 (November 1993).

Rosenberg, Debra, and Evan Thomas. "I didn't do anything." *Newsweek* 130, no. 19 (November 10, 1997): 60.

Rothschild, M.A., and V. Schneider. "'Terminal Burrowing Behavior'—A Phenomenon of Lethal Hypothermia." *International Journal of Legal Medicine* 107, no. 5 (September 1995): 250–56.

Ruan, Jesse, and Priya Prasad. "The Effects of Skull Thickness Variations on Human Head Dynamic Impact Responses." SAE Journal, November 2001. http://www.sae.org/technicalpapers/2001-22-0018 (accessed July 23, 2009).

Sachs, Jessica Snyder. "Drug Cartels Raise the Game for the Mule Trackers." *Popular Science* 264, no. 6 (June 1, 2004): 38.

Saferstein, Richard. *Criminalistics: An Introduction to Forensic Science.* 7th ed. Upper Saddle River, NJ: Prentice Hall, 2001.

"Safety: Natural Gas Safety." Power House. http://www.powerhousetv.com/stellent2/groups/public/documents/pub/phtv_sa_ga_000340.hcsp (accessed August 22, 2004).

Schultz, Donald O. *Criminal Investigation Techniques.* Houston: Gulf Publishing Company, 1978.

Schwartz, R.H., R. Milteer, and M.A. LeBeau. "Drug-Facilitated Sexual Assault ('Date Rape')." *Southern Medical Journal* 93, no. 6 (June 2000): 558–61.

Shields, L.B., D.M. Hunsaker, and J.C. Hunsaker, III. "Autoerotic Asphyxia: Part I." *American Journal of Forensic Medicine and Pathology* 26, no. 1 (March 2005): 45–52.

Simpson, David M., and Steven Stehr Stern. "Victim Management and Identification After the World Trade Center Collapse." 2003. http://www.colorado.edu/hazards/sp/sp39/sept11book_ch4_simpson.pdf (accessed August 1, 2005).

Sivaloganathan, S. "Paraodoxical Undressing and Hypothermia." *Medicine, Science, and the Law* 26, no. 3 (July 1986): 225–29.

Smart, Reginald G. "Cocaine." In *Forbidden Highs: The Nature, Treatment, and Prevention of Illicit Drug Abuse,* by Reginald G. Smart, 79–86. Toronto: Addiction Research Foundation, 1983.

Smith, Carlton. *Cold Blooded.* New York: St. Martin's Paperbacks, 2004.

Smith, Cathy. *Chasing the Dragon.* Toronto: Key Porter Books, 1984.

Smock, W.S. "Recognition of Pattern Injuries in Domestic Violence Victims." In *Encyclopedia of Forensic Sciences,* Vol. 1, edited by Pekka J. Saukko and Geoffrey C. Knupfer, 384–91. San Diego: Academic Press, 2000.

"The Smoking of Heroin in Hong Kong." United Nations Office on Drugs and Crime Bulletin on Narcotics. http://www.unodc.org/unodc/en/bulletin/bulletin_1958-01-01_3_page003.html (accessed August 11, 2004).

"So You Want to be a Medical Detective?" National Association of Medical Examiners (NAME). http://www.thename.org/medical_detective.htm (accessed June 24, 2004).

Soonprasert, Kittipong. "Thai Coroner Seeks Cause of David Carradine's Death." Reuters. http://www.reuters.com/article/topNews/idUSTRE5334TM20090605?pageNumber=2&virtualBrandChannel=0&sp=true (accessed June 5, 2009).

Spitz, Werner U. "Selected Procedures at Autopsy." In *Medicolegal Investigation of Death: Guidelines for the Application of Pathology to Crime Investigation,* edited by Werner U. Spitz and Russell S. Fisher, 590–603. 2nd ed. Springfield, IL: Charles C. Thomas, 1980.

"Spy Poisoning: 300 Seek Radiation Tests." CNN.com.World, November 26, 2006. http://www.cnn.com/2006/WORLD/europe/11/26/uk.spy.ap/index.html?eref=rss_top stories (accessed December 2, 2006).

Starrs, James E. *A Voice for the Dead: A Forensic Investigator's Pursuit of the Truth in the Grave.* New York: Berkeley Books, 2005.

Stephens, B.G., J.M. Jentzen, S. Karch, D.C. Mash, and C.V. Wetli. "Criteria for the Interpretation of Cocaine Levels in Human Biological Samples and Their Relation to the Cause of Death." *American Journal of Forensic Medicine and Pathology* 25, no. 1 (March 2004): 1–10.

"Steps of an Autopsy." Death: The Last Taboo. http://www.deathonline.net/what happens/autopsysteps.cfm (accessed July 23, 2009).

"The Story of Cocaine." California Narcotic Officers' Association. http://www.cnoa.org/N-04.pdf (accessed July 15, 2004).

Stover, Dawn. "Was It Murder?" *Popular Science* 254, no. 4 (April 1999): 78–81.

Straight, Richard C., and James L. Glenn. "Human Fatalities Caused by Venomous Animals in Utah, 1900–90." *Great Basin Naturalist* 53, no. 4 (1993): 390–94.

Strang, J., P. Griffiths, and M. Gossop. "Heroin Smoking by 'Chasing the Dragon': Origins and History." *Addiction* 92, no. 6 (June 1997): 673–83.

Sulek, Julia Prodis. "Hypothermia Claimed James Kim." *Oakland Tribune*, Friday, December 8, 2006. http://www.findarticles.com/p/articles/mi_qn4176/is_20061208/ai_n16896899 (accessed December 30, 2006).

Sullivan, Terry, and Peter T. Maiken. *Killer Clown: The John Wayne Gacy Murders.* New York: Pinnacle Books, 1983.

Taber, Stephen Welton. *Fire Ants.* College Station, TX: Texas A & M University Press, 2000.

Tarabar, A.F., and L.S. Nelson. "The Gamma-hydroxybutyrate Withdrawal Syndrome." *Toxicological Reviews* 23, no. 1 (2004): 45–49.

Taylor, George E., Jr., and Clifford L. Linedecker. *Club Fed: A True Story of Life, Lies, and Crime in the Federal Witness Protection Program.* New York: Avon Books, 1998.

Taylor, Purcell, Jr. "Crack." In *Substance Abuse: Pharmacologic and Developmental Perspectives,* by Purcell Taylor, Jr., 59–61. Springfield, IL: Charles C. Thomas, 1998.

Temple, John. *Deadhouse: Life in a Coroner's Office.* Jackson, MS: University Press of Mississippi, 2005.

Teresa, Vincent, and Thomas C. Renner. *My Life in the Mafia.* Greenwich, CT: Fawcett Publications, 1973.

Thomas, Bob. *Golden Boy: The Untold Story of William Holden.* New York: St. Martin's Press, 1983.

Thomas, Gordon, and Martin Dillon. *Robert Maxwell Israel's Superspy: The Life and Murder of a Media Mogul.* New York: Carroll & Graf Publishers, 2002.

"Thomas J. Shepardson." Disaster Mortuary Operational Response Team. http://www.dmort.org/DNPages/In_memory_obit.htm (accessed November 30, 2005a).

"Thomas J. Shepardson." National Obituary Archive. http://www.arrangeonline.com/obituary.asp?obituaryid=67380672 (accessed November 30, 2005b).

Thompson, Robert L., William W. Manders, and William R. Cowan. "Postmortem Findings of the Victims of the Jonestown Tragedy." *Journal of Forensic Sciences* 32, no. 2 (March 1987): 433–43.

Timmermans, Stefan. *Postmortem: How Medical Examiners Explain Suspicious Deaths.* Chicago: University of Chicago Press, 2006.

Travers, Bridget, editor. *World of Invention.* Detroit: Gale Research, 1994.

Turvey, Brent E. *Criminal Profiling: An Introduction to Behavioral Evidence Analysis.* 2nd ed. San Diego: Academic Press, 2002.

U.S. National Drug Intelligence Center. National Drug Threat Assessment 2005: Heroin. www.usdoj.gov.ndic/pubs11/12620/heroin.htm (accessed July 23, 2009).

U.S. Patent 6395234—Sample Cassette Having Utility for Histological Processing of Tissue Samples. PatientStorm. http://www.patientstorm.us/patents6395234/description.html (accessed July 24, 2009).

Van Nostrand's Encyclopedia of Chemistry. 2005. s.v. "Chromatography."

Vanezis, P. "Interpreting Bruises at Necropsy." *Journal of Clinical Pathology* 54 (2001): 348–55.

Varetto, Lorenzo, and Ombretta Curto. "Long Persistence of Rigor Mortis at Constant Low Temperature." *Forensic Science International* 147, no. 1 (2005): 31–34.

Vass, Arpad A. "Beyond the Grave: Understanding Human Decomposition." *Microbiology Today* 28 (November 2001): 190–92.

Villa, Peter D. "Midfacial Complications of Prolonged Cocaine Snort." *Journal of the Canadian Dental Association* 65 (1999): 218–23.

Walsh, Tom. "Gene Codes Scales Down Massive Victim ID Project: Software for DNA Matching Took Technology to New Levels." *Detroit Free Press*, Thursday, September 9, 2004. www.freep.com (accessed January 19, 2005).

Wecht, Cyril. Telephone interview by Tia L. Lindstrom, July 15, 2009.

Wecht, Cyril, Mark Curriden, and Benjamin Wecht. *Cause of Death*. New York: Onyx, 1994.

Wecht, Cyril, Greg Saitz, and Mark Curriden. *Mortal Evidence: The Forensics Behind Nine Shocking Cases*. Amherst, NY: Prometheus Books, 2003.

Wecht, Cyril H, general editor. *Crime Scene Investigation: Crack the Case with Real-Life Experts*. Pleasantville, NY: Reader's Digest, 2004.

Wedin, B., L. Vanggaard, and J. Hirvonen. "'Paradoxical Undressing' in Fatal Hypothermia." *Journal of Forensic Sciences* 24, no. 3 (July 1979): 543–53.

Wesselius, C.L., and R. Bally. "A Male with Autoerotic Asphyxia Syndrome." *American Journal of Forensic Medicine and Pathology* 4, no. 4 (December 1983): 341–44.

Wetli, C.V., and R.E. Mittleman. "The 'Body Packer Syndrome': Toxicity Following Ingestion of Illicit Drugs Packaged for Transportation." *Journal of Forensic Sciences* 26, no. 3 (July 1981): 492–500.

Weyand, Ernest H. "Sudden, Unexplained Infant Death Investigations." *FBI Law Enforcement Bulletin* 73, no. 3 (March 2004): 10–15.

"What Is Mass Spectrometry?" American Society for Mass Spectrometry: Education. December 1, 2001. http://www.asms.org/whatisms/p3.html (accessed July 13, 2005).

"What Is Rigor Mortis?" Australian Museum Online. 2003. www.deathonline.net/decomposition/body_changes/rigor_mortis_htm (accessed February 11, 2007).

"While Strongly Favoring Burial in the Earth, in 1963 the Catholic Church for the First Time Permitted the Practice of Cremation." *First Things* 159 (January 1, 2006): 70.

"Whitewater: The Foster Report." 1998 washingtonpost.com. http://www.washingtonpost.com/wp-srv/politics/special/whitewater/docs/fosteri.htm (accessed December 26, 2006).

"Whittaker, D.K. "An Introduction to Forensic Dentistry." *Quintessence International* 25, no. 10 (October 1994): 723–30.

William Holden. http://www.findadeath.com (accessed August 23, 2004).

"William Holden." High-Profile Autopsy Files. http://www.celebritycollectables.com/cgi-bin/ezshopper/loadpage.cgi?user_id=97039&file=autopsy.htm (accessed August 31, 2004).

Williams, David A. "Bitemark Analysis Is a Critical Component of Forensic Odontology." *Forensic Nurse* (January/February 2003). http://www.forensicnursemag.com/articles/311feat5.html (accessed December 26, 2005).

Wolcott, John H., and Charles A. Hanson. "Summary of the Means Used to Positively Identify the American Victims in the Canary Islands Crash." *Aviation, Space, and Environmental Medicine* 51, no. 9 (September 1980): 1034–35.

Wolf, Marvin J., and Katherine Mader. *Fallen Angels: Chronicles of L.A. Crime and Mystery.* New York: Facts on File Publications, 1986.

Wollina, U., H.J. Kammler, N. Hesselbarth, B. Mock, and H. Bosseckert. "Ecstasy Pimples—A New Facial Dermatosis." *Dermatology* (Basel, Switzerland) 197, no. 2 (1998): 171–73.

"Woman Accused in Murder Hangs Herself." *Milwaukee Journal Sentinel,* Monday, April 1, 2002. http://www.findarticles.com/p/articles/mi_qn4196/is_20020401/ai_ n10776406 (accessed November 18, 2006).

Yanai, O., and J. Hiss. "Cocaine 'Mules.'" *Harefuah* 136, no. 3 (February 1, 1999): 190–93 and 255.

Yoo, In-Sung. "Autopsy Minus the Scalpel." *USA Today,* Tuesday, March 23, 2004. http://web.ebscohost.com/ehost/delivery?vid=120&hid=18&sid=006e50c6-2ad1-4a 09-b13. . . (accessed February 14, 2007).

Young, Robyn V, editor. *World of Chemistry.* Detroit: Gale Group, 2000.

Zaki, S.A., and R. Hanzlick. "Gunshot Wound with Asphalt Related Pseudo-Soot, Pseudo-Tattooing, and Pseudo-Scorching." *Journal of Forensic Sciences* 32, no. 4 (July 1987): 1136–40.

INDEX

About the Authors

JOHN J. MILETICH writes primarily about psychopathology, true crime, and substance abuse. His previous books include *Homicide Investigation: An Introduction*. He is a graduate of the University of Alberta and the University of Western Ontario.

TIA LAURA LINDSTROM is a freelance writer who writes on health and medical issues. She is a graduate of the University of British Columbia.

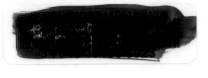
Introduction to the work of a medical
examiner : from death scene to autopsy
suite / John J. Miletich and Tia Laura
Lindstrom ; foreword by Cyril H. Wecht.